NO HORMONE IMBALANCES

A MASTER HERBALIST'S GUIDE FOR BALANCING WOMEN'S HORMONE HEALTH THROUGH HERBAL REMEDIES AND HOLISTIC HEALING

A comprehensive and practical guide for women looking to take control and balance their hormonal health Herbally

APRIL HEATH-WHITE , M.S., B.S., A.A.

Copyright © 2023 by April Heath-White , M.S., B.S., A.A.

Disclaimer

Disclaimer Statements made in this eBook regarding herbal supplements and herbs have yet to be evaluated by the food and drug administration. This information has not been evaluated by the U.S. Food and Drug Administration. The information presented in this book is provided for informational purposes only; it is not meant to substitute for medical advice or diagnosis provided by your physician or other medical professionals. The Herbs in this Book are not intended to treat, cure, or prevent any illness or disease. If you have or suspect a medical problem, contact your physician or health care provider. Always consult your physician or health care provider before using any herbal products, especially if you are pregnant or have a medical problem. The images of herbs, foods and other images included in this Book were obtained from free sources on the internet. While we have made every effort to ensure that these images are used in compliance with the licensing terms, we cannot guarantee their accuracy or authenticity. If you believe that any of the images used in this Book infringe on your intellectual property rights, please contact us immediately, and we will take appropriate action. Also, while the information in this Book is accurate to the best of our knowledge, we cannot be liable for any damages that may result from using this information. This Book is intended for informational purposes only, and we recommend that you consult a qualified healthcare professional before using any of the herbal remedies discussed in this Book.

TABLE OF CONTENTS

About The Author 6
My struggles with Hormone Imbalance 8
What is Hormonal Imbalance 13
Signs & Symptoms of Hormone Imbalances 20
What is Herbal Medicine 24

Herb 1: Black Cohosh Herb 32
 Case Studies on Black Cohosh 34
 Recipe 1: Black Cohosh Herbal Tea 35
 Recipe 2: Black Cohosh Smoothie 36
 Recipe 3: Black Cohosh Juice 37

Herb 2: Dong Quai Herb 38
 Case Studies on Dong Quai 40
 Recipe 1: Dong Quai Herbal Tea 42
 Recipe 2: Dong Quai Smoothie 43
 Recipe 3: Dong Quai Juice 44

Herb 3: Chaste Tree Berry (Vitex) Herb 45
 Case Studies on Chaste Tree Berry (Vitex) 47
 Recipe 1: Chaste Tree Berry Smoothie 48
 Recipe 2: Chaste Tree Berry Juice 49
 Recipe 3: Chaste Tree Berry Herbal Tea 50

Herb 4: Red Clover Herb 52
 Case Studies on Red Clover 54
 Recipe 1: Red Clover Smoothie 55

Recipe 2: Red Clover Juice 56
Recipe 3: Red Clover Herbal Tea 57

Herb 5: Sanguisorba Officinalis (Dog Blood) Herb 59
Case Studies on Sanguisorba Officinalis (Dog Blood) Herb . . . 61
Recipe 1: Sanguisorba Officinalis Smoothie. 62
Recipe 2: Sanguisorba Officinalis Juice. 63
Recipe 3: Sanguisorba Officinalis Herbal Tea. 64

Herb 6: Evening Primrose Herb. 66
Case Studies on Evening Primrose. 68
Recipe 1: Evening Primrose Herbal Tea. 69
Recipe 2: Evening Primrose Smoothie with Pineapple,
Mango, and Coconut Water 70
Recipe 3: Strawberry Evening Primrose Smoothie. 71
Recipe 4: Evening Primrose juice with kale, spinach,
cucumber, green apples, and ginger. 72

Herb 7: Maca Root Herb 73
Case Studies on Maca Root 75
Recipe 1: Maca Root "Strong Back" Smoothie. 76
Recipe 2: Nutritious Maca Root Juice. 77
Recipe 3: Maca Root Herbal Tea 78

Herb 8: Red Raspberry Leaf (Rubus idaeus) Herb 80
Case Studies on Red Raspberry Leaf Case 82
Recipe 1: Red Raspberry Leaf Herbal Tea 83
Recipe 2: Red Raspberry Smoothie 84
Recipe 3: Refreshing and healthy Red Raspberry Juice. 85

Herb 9: Wild Yam (Dioscorea Villosa) Herb 86
Case Studies on Wild Yam 88
Recipe 1: Wild Yam Herbal Tea 89

Recipe 2: Wild Yam Smoothie 89
Recipe 3: Wild Yam Juice 90

Bonus Herb #1: Burdock root (Arctium lappa). 92
Case Studies on Burdock Root. 94
Bonus Recipe 1: Burdock Root Herbal Tea (Blood Cleanser) . . 95
Bonus Recipe 2: Herbal Tea Potent Support
Formula to Balance the Hormone. 96
Bonus Recipe 3: Delicious Burdock Root Smoothie. 97
Bonus Recipe 4: Delicious Burdock Root Juice 98

Bonus Herb #2: Sea Moss (Chondrus crispus) AKA Irish Moss . . 100
Case Studies on SEA MOSS 102
Sea Moss Gel Recipe 104
Sea Moss Bonus Smoothie Recipe # 1 105
Sea Moss Bonus Smoothie Recipe # 2 106

Eating the Right Foods, Fruits,
and Vegetables for Hormone Imbalances 108
Recipe 1: Quinoa and Kale Salad 112
Recipe 3: Lentil Soup 114
Recipe 4: Roasted Sweet Potato and Brussels Sprouts 116
Recipe 5: Chocolate Avocado Pudding. 117

Exercises for Hormone Imbalances. 119
Sleep and Hormone Balance and
Hydration and Hormone Balance. 125

ABOUT THE AUTHOR

April Heath-White

In the picturesque fishing village of Rocky Point, Clarendon, Jamaica, a young girl named April Heath-White, known by her pen name Israel, began her extraordinary journey. From an early age, April possessed a deep curiosity and an unyielding determination to conquer any challenges that came her way.

At 14, April embarked on a new adventure, leaving behind the familiar shores of her homeland to start a new life in the United States. It was a daunting transition, but April's indomitable spirit and thirst for knowledge propelled her. She quickly adapted to her new surroundings and excelled in her studies, graduating from high school with honors.

Driven by her innate passion for storytelling, April pursued her dreams in journalism. She embarked on a path of learning and growth, earning an associate degree in Broadcasting Journalism. However, her journey was far from over. April's insatiable curiosity led her to explore another realm that captivated her heart—health and wellness.

Fueling her passion, April began a new educational pursuit, earning a bachelor's in business project management from the esteemed City College of Fort Lauderdale. But that was not enough. Her deep desire to understand the intricacies of herbal medicine and its profound impact on human health beckoned her toward a new chapter in her life.

Undeterred by the challenges ahead, April pursued a master's degree in Herbal Medicine with a specialization in Nutrition from The American

College of Healthcare & Science (ACHS) in Portland, Oregon. Her dedication and commitment to her studies paid off, and in June 2020, she proudly became a Master Herbalist.

April's journey did not stop there. She is an herbalist, entrepreneur, interviewer, and devoted vegan for over a decade. Her quest for knowledge and unwavering passion for helping others led her to assist clients with various ailments and diseases. She tirelessly sought new herbs and explored the realm of vegan foods, embracing the power of natural remedies and nutrition.

Amidst her busy life, April found solace and joy in the simplicity of life's pleasures. She relished exercising on the sun-kissed beaches, finding inspiration in the rhythm of crashing waves. She treasured the precious moments spent with her loving husband, cherished family, and dear friends.

April's wealth of experience, knowledge, and unwavering dedication to promoting health and wellness made her the perfect author for this book on balancing hormones in women. Her unique blend of journalistic prowess, herbal expertise, and personal journey gives her a profound understanding of women's challenges in achieving hormonal balance.

Through her book, April aims to share her wisdom, empowering women to take control of their health and well-being. Her journey, filled with resilience, triumphs, and a deep passion for natural healing, is a beacon of hope for all those seeking harmony in their hormonal journey.

So, join April Heath-White, a woman of many talents and a guiding light in the world of herbal medicine, as she unveils the secrets to balancing hormones and unlocking the path to radiant health for women everywhere.

MY STRUGGLES WITH HORMONE IMBALANCE

Once upon a time, I was no different from the women I now strive to help. My journey with hormone imbalances was riddled with pain, frustration, and a desperate search for relief.

Fibroids, cysts, heavy and painful menstrual cycles, vomiting, anxiety – the list seemed endless. In the depths of my struggle with hormone imbalances, I faced a daunting obstacle that forever altered the trajectory of my life. It was a time when my faith in traditional medicine was tested, and I yearned for a glimmer of hope to guide me through the darkness.

The journey began innocently enough as I sought help from a well-intentioned medical doctor who prescribed birth control to alleviate my symptoms. Little did I know that this harmless solution would soon unleash a storm of unforeseen consequences upon my body.

Months passed, and I was caught in a tumultuous whirlwind of pain, discomfort, and mounting frustration. My periods became more erratic, and a persistent heaviness settled deep within me. Unbeknownst to me, birth control, intended to alleviate my suffering and balance my hormones, had become the catalyst for a harrowing journey ahead.

Then, one fateful day, I discovered that I was pregnant. Hope mingled with trepidation as I eagerly anticipated the arrival of my new life. However, the universe had a different plan in store for me. In a cruel twist of fate, the little life growing within me had nestled itself outside the protective walls of the Fallopian tube.

An **ectopic pregnancy**, they called it – a scary situation where the life I carried was in grave danger, and so was my own. As the weeks passed, the baby grew, but not where it should have been. Desperation set in as I grappled with excruciating pain and an unrelenting sense of helplessness.

The moment I arrived when my only recourse was an emergency surgery, a life-or-death race against time. With every passing moment, the risk grew more fantastic, and the walls of despair closed in. In that operating room, the weight of my ordeal bore down on me as I surrendered to the skilled hands of the medical team.

The surgery was successful, but the scars left behind were not just physical. They cut deep into the core of my being, leaving me grappling with an overwhelming sense of loss and grief. The weight of my pain pressed upon me, dragging me into depression.

The aftermath of my ectopic pregnancy surgery led me down a treacherous path filled with confusion, frustration, and a desperate search for answers.

As I sought solace and healing at the Florida Medical Center, I placed my trust in the medical experts who, unfortunately, proved to be ill-equipped to navigate the complexities of my unique situation. Unbeknownst to me, their lack of understanding and experience would lead to a series of fateful decisions that would forever alter the course of my reproductive journey.

In their attempts to address the issue, the doctors decided to tie my remaining fallopian tube. Their intentions, though well-meaning, brought about unintended consequences that further compounded my struggles. With my dreams of conceiving a child hanging precariously in the balance, I was entangled in a web of uncertainty and anguish.

Determined to find a solution, I embarked on a desperate quest to untangle the knot that had been tied within me. The medical journey that ensued was fraught with uncertainty and disappointment. I underwent not just one but two surgeries in a valiant attempt to restore the functionality of my fallopian tube. Alas, despite their best efforts, the outcome remained unchanged. The doctors confessed that the chances of successfully untying the knot were no more than a 50-50 gamble.

My heart sank as I grappled with the harsh reality of my situation. The weight of infertility pressed upon me, threatening to shatter the fragments of hope that still clung to my spirit. In these moments of despair, I realized I could no longer place the entirety of my faith in the hands of conventional medicine alone.

In the depths of my despair, I discovered a glimmer of hope in the form of herbal medicine. Driven by a burning desire for change, I underwent a profound personal transformation.

Enrolling in a master's degree program, I immersed myself in the world of herbs, determined to find solace within their embrace. And so, with trepidation and a newfound resolve, I began my healing journey.

To my astonishment, I experienced a shift like never before within a month of embracing herbal remedies. My flow normalized, the torment of vomiting ceased, and the once-pervasive pain, fibroids, cysts, and anxiety diminished to a whisper. All my suffering dissipated three months later, and medical professionals confirmed that my hormones were finally balanced, and fallopian tube untied.

This life-altering experience kindled a passion within me. I felt compelled to share the power of herbal medicine with other women, to offer them the chance to regain control over their hormones and lives. In its infinite wisdom, nature had provided us with a bountiful arsenal of remedies, and I became determined to unlock their secrets and share them with the world.

Thus, I embarked on a mission to become a Master Herbalist – a beacon of hope for those facing the same struggles I had endured for far too long. Through my practice, I witnessed firsthand the transformative effects of natural remedies on women's hormone health. Their stories of triumph and healing fueled my dedication to spreading knowledge and empowering others to tap into the incredible potential of herbal medicine.

And now, I invite you to join me on this journey of discovery and empowerment. Within the pages of this book, I will impart valuable insights and tools that will enable you to reclaim your hormone health and transform your overall well-being.

Drawing upon years of research and practical experience, I have formulated herbal supplements and tinctures to address an array of ailments and diseases, including the intricate web of hormone imbalances. Witnessing the remarkable results achieved by countless women who have embraced these remedies, I am filled with a sense of purpose and renewed determination.

This book serves as a comprehensive guide, illuminating the intricacies of hormone imbalances in women – an issue that plagues millions worldwide. Together, we will explore the rich history and multifaceted benefits of herbal medicine and supplements in achieving hormonal balance and alleviating symptoms. Through fascinating case studies, we will delve into the remarkable healing properties of popular herbs such as Black cohosh, Chasteberry, and red raspberry leaf, unveiling their potential to regulate and restore harmony within your hormones.

But hormonal balance extends beyond herbal medicine alone. Recognizing the holistic nature of our bodies, we will also explore the profound impact of lifestyle changes on hormone regulation. From tailored exercise plans to delectable recipes featuring hormone-friendly ingredients, this book offers practical guidance on nurturing your body through movement and nourishment.

Furthermore, you will find an exquisite collection of recipes with the ingredients and instructions needed to craft delightful herbal teas, refreshing smoothies, and rejuvenating juices – each designed to optimize hormone balance and invigorate your well-being.

Lastly, I will share my journey – a tale of resilience, discovery, and unwavering determination. Through my triumphs and tribulations, you will witness the transformative power of embracing natural remedies and reclaiming control over your hormone health.

This book is a beacon of hope for women seeking understanding, support, and actionable steps toward managing their hormone imbalances. Together, let us embark on self-discovery, empowerment, and renewed vitality. Welcome to a world where balance and harmony await – women reign supreme over their hormones and live their lives to the fullest.

▶ WHAT IS HORMONAL IMBALANCE

Hormone imbalance is an abnormality in the body's production, distribution, or action of hormones. Hormones are chemical messengers that regulate various physiological processes, such as growth and development, metabolism, reproduction, and mood. When hormones are not produced, distributed, or utilized correctly, it can lead to various health problems, including hormone imbalances.

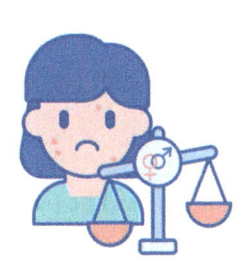

Hormonal imbalance is a disruption or irregularity in the levels or functioning of hormones in the body. Hormones are chemical messengers that play vital roles in regulating various bodily functions and processes. The endocrine glands produce them and maintain balance and harmony within the body.

The endocrine glands are a collection of glands in the body that produce and secrete hormones directly into the bloodstream. These glands regulate and control various bodily functions, maintain homeostasis, and coordinate communication between different organs and tissues.

Here are some vital endocrine glands and their functions:

Pituitary Gland: At the base of the brain, the pituitary gland is called the "master gland" because it controls the functions of many other endocrine glands. It secretes hormones that regulate growth, reproduction, metabolism, and water balance.

Thyroid Gland: in the neck, the thyroid gland produces hormones that regulate metabolism, body temperature, and energy levels. It also plays a crucial role in growth and development.

Adrenal Glands: on top of the kidneys, the adrenal glands produce hormones such as cortisol, which helps manage stress and regulate metabolism, and adrenaline, which triggers the body's "fight or flight" response.

Pancreas: The pancreas has both endocrine and exocrine functions. The endocrine part produces insulin and glucagon, which regulate blood sugar levels and metabolism.

Ovaries: In females, the ovaries produce estrogen and progesterone, which are involved in reproductive functions, menstrual cycle regulation, and pregnancy.

Testes: In males, the testes produce testosterone, responsible for male sexual characteristics, fertility, and reproductive functions.

Pineal Gland: In the brain, the pineal gland produces the hormone melatonin, which helps regulate the sleep-wake cycle and circadian rhythms.

Parathyroid Glands: Located near the thyroid gland, the parathyroid glands produce parathyroid hormone (PTH), which regulates calcium and phosphorus levels in the body.

These endocrine glands release hormones into the bloodstream, allowing them to travel to target cells or organs throughout the body. Hormones act as chemical messengers, binding to specific receptors on cells and triggering various physiological responses. They help regulate growth, metabolism, sexual function, mood, sleep, and other processes necessary for overall health and well-being.

The endocrine system works in coordination with other systems in the body, such as the nervous system, to maintain balance and ensure the proper functioning of the body's cells and organs.

Any disruption or dysfunction within the endocrine glands can lead to hormonal imbalances and various health problems.

The relationship between the endocrine system and the nervous system is intricate and vital for the proper functioning of the human body. Throughout history, scientists and medical experts have been fascinated by the interconnectedness of these two systems, unraveling their complex interactions and uncovering their profound impact on overall health and well-being.

The story of the endocrine and nervous systems begins in ancient times, with early civilizations recognizing the significance of glands and their secretions. Ancient Egyptians, for instance, believed that the heart, not the brain, was the center of intelligence and emotions. It was not until the time of Hippocrates, the ancient Greek physician often referred to as the "Father of Medicine," that the importance of the brain and its connection to other bodily functions started to be recognized.

Fast forward to the 17th and 18th centuries when anatomists and scientists made significant discoveries about the nervous system. Thomas Willis, an English physician, conducted groundbreaking research on the brain and its functions, laying the foundation for our understanding of the nervous system. Willis coined the term "neurology" and identified the connection between the brain and the rest of the body through nerves.

Simultaneously, advancements have been made in our understanding of the endocrine system. Claude Bernard, a French physiologist, is known for his work on the body's internal environment and the concept of homeostasis. He recognized the importance of glands and their secretions in maintaining the body's balance and coined the term "milieu Inférieur," which later influenced the development of endocrinology.

In the early 20th century, the connection between the endocrine and nervous systems became more apparent. British physiologists William Bayliss and Ernest Starling discovered a hormone called secretin, which stimulated pancreatic secretions. This groundbreaking finding highlighted the communication between the gastrointestinal tract and hormonal signals, linking the endocrine system to digestive processes.

Further advancements in the mid-20th century shed light on the intricate relationship between the endocrine and nervous systems. The discovery of the hypothalamus as a crucial brain region regulating hormone release was a significant milestone. Geoffrey Harris, a British neuroendocrinologist, elucidated the role of the hypothalamus in controlling the pituitary gland, often referred to as the "master gland" due to its control over other endocrine glands.

Through extensive research and scientific discoveries, we now understand that the endocrine and nervous systems work in tandem to maintain homeostasis and regulate various physiological processes. The hypothalamus in the brain plays a significant role in connecting these two systems. It releases hormones that stimulate or inhibit the release of hormones from the pituitary gland, which, in turn, regulates other endocrine glands throughout the body.

The intricate relationship between the endocrine and nervous systems extends beyond the hypothalamus-pituitary axis. Nerve signals can also directly influence the release of hormones from certain glands, such as the adrenal glands. For example, stress triggers the release of stress hormones like cortisol by activating the hypothalamic-pituitary-adrenal (H.P.A.) axis, highlighting the collaboration between the two systems.

This historical journey of discovery and scientific progress has deepened our understanding of the interplay between the endocrine and nervous systems. Today, we recognize that hormones released by the endocrine glands act as chemical messengers, transmitting signals throughout the body. At the same time, the nervous system uses electrical impulses and neurotransmitters to communicate information rapidly.

In summary, the relationship between the endocrine and nervous systems involves intricate coordination and communication. The evolution of our understanding of these systems has been a testament to the curiosity and dedication of scientists and researchers throughout history. Their

discoveries have paved the way for a comprehensive understanding of how these systems regulate bodily functions and maintain optimal health.

Several Vitamins and Minerals also play crucial roles in hormone synthesis and regulation. Here are some key ones:

Vitamin D: Known as the "sunshine vitamin," vitamin D is vital in hormone regulation. It supports the production and function of various hormones, including insulin, estrogen, progesterone, and testosterone. Adequate vitamin D levels are essential for maintaining hormonal balance.

Vitamin B6: This vitamin is involved in the synthesis and metabolism of various hormones, including serotonin, dopamine, and melatonin. It also supports the production of progesterone, estrogen, and testosterone.

Vitamin C: As an antioxidant, vitamin C helps protect the body against oxidative stress and supports the adrenal glands, which produce stress hormones like cortisol. It also aids in the production of progesterone and estrogen.

Vitamin E: This vitamin acts as an antioxidant and supports the health of the reproductive system. It is involved in producing and regulating hormones, including estrogen and progesterone.

Magnesium: Magnesium plays a vital role in hormone synthesis and balance. It supports the production of progesterone and helps regulate insulin levels. Additionally, magnesium aids in the conversion of inactive thyroid hormone (T4) into active thyroid hormone (T3).

Zinc: Zinc is involved in the synthesis and regulation of various hormones, including insulin, thyroid hormones, and sex hormones like estrogen and testosterone. It also supports proper immune function and aids in the metabolism of hormones.

Iodine: Iodine is essential for producing thyroid hormones, which regulate metabolism and growth. Adequate iodine levels are necessary for optimal thyroid function and hormonal balance.

Selenium: Selenium is an important mineral for thyroid health and function. It supports the conversion of T4 to T3, the active form of thyroid hormone. Selenium also acts as an antioxidant, protecting the thyroid gland from oxidative damage.

Iron: Iron is necessary for producing hemoglobin, which carries oxygen to cells. It also supports the production and function of several hormones, including those involved in energy metabolism and growth.

These vitamins and minerals are found in various Herbal supplements, foods, including fruits, vegetables, whole grains, legumes, nuts, seeds, and lean proteins. A balanced diet incorporating these nutrient-rich foods can support optimal hormone synthesis and regulation.

SIGNS & SYMPTOMS OF HORMONE IMBALANCES

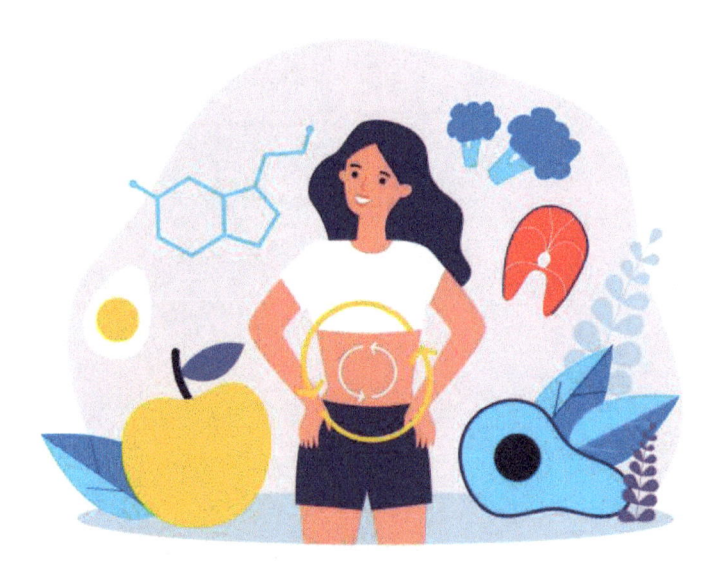

It is important to note that not all women will experience all these symptoms and that they can vary in severity depending on the individual and the specific hormonal imbalance. Symptoms of hormone imbalances in women vary depending on the type and severity of the condition. Some common signs and symptoms include:

In a healthy state, hormones work together in a delicate balance, acting as signals communicating with different organs and tissues to regulate functions such as metabolism, growth and development, reproduction, mood, sleep, and energy levels. However, when there is a disturbance in this balance, it can lead to hormonal imbalances.

Hormonal imbalances can occur due to several factors, including:

Stress: Chronic stress can disrupt the production and balance of hormones in the body, particularly the stress hormone cortisol. This can have cascading effects on other hormones.

Age and Life Stages: Hormonal fluctuations are common during certain life stages, such as puberty, pregnancy, and menopause. These transitions can cause temporary imbalances and associated symptoms.

Medical Conditions: Certain medical conditions, such as polycystic ovary syndrome (PCOS), thyroid disorders, diabetes, and adrenal disorders, can affect hormone levels and lead to imbalances.

Lifestyle Factors: Poor diet, lack of exercise, inadequate sleep, and exposure to environmental toxins can all contribute to hormonal imbalances.

Medications and Treatments: Certain medications, such as hormonal contraceptives or hormone replacement therapy, can influence hormone levels and potentially disrupt the natural balance.

Implications of hormone imbalance for women's health can manifest in several ways:

Menstrual Irregularities: Hormone imbalances can cause irregular, heavy, or absent periods, disrupting the natural menstrual cycle and affecting fertility.

Polycystic Ovary Syndrome (PCOS): PCOS is a hormonal disorder characterized by elevated levels of androgens (male hormones) and imbalances in insulin. It can lead to symptoms such as irregular periods, ovarian cysts, acne, excessive hair growth, and weight gain.

Menopause and Perimenopause: During menopause, hormone levels, particularly estrogen and progesterone, decline. This transition can cause symptoms like hot flashes, night sweats, mood swings, vaginal dryness, and changes in bone density.

Thyroid Disorders: Imbalances in thyroid hormones regulating metabolism can lead to hypothyroidism (underactive thyroid) or hyperthyroidism (overactive thyroid). These disorders can affect energy levels, weight, mood, and well-being.

Reproductive Health Issues: Hormone imbalances can contribute to fertility problems, including ovulation disorders and hormonal issues affecting the reproductive system. They can also impact pregnancy outcomes and increase the risk of conditions like endometriosis or uterine fibroids.

Mood Disorders: Hormone imbalances, particularly fluctuations in estrogen and progesterone, can contribute to mood disorders such as depression, anxiety, irritability, and mood swings.

Bone Health: Hormones like estrogen are vital in maintaining bone density. Imbalances can increase the risk of osteoporosis and bone fractures.

Metabolic and Weight Issues: Hormone imbalances, especially insulin resistance and imbalances in leptin and ghrelin (hunger-regulating hormones), can contribute to weight gain, difficulty losing weight, and metabolic disorders like diabetes.

Acne: Hormone imbalances can cause acne breakouts, particularly around the chin and jawline.

Hair loss: Changes in hormone levels can cause hair loss or thinning, particularly in women experiencing menopause.

Brain fog or difficulty concentrating: Changes in hormone levels may lead to problems doing tasks or jobs.

Hot flashes and night sweats: These symptoms are commonly associated with menopause but can also occur due to hormonal imbalances at other stages of life.

Vaginal dryness: Hormonal changes can cause vaginal dryness, leading to discomfort during sexual activity.

Sleep disturbances: Hormone imbalances can disrupt sleep patterns, leading to difficulty falling or staying asleep.

Decreased sex drive: Changes in hormone levels can lead to a decrease in sex drive or low libido.

Changes in appetite or cravings: Changes in hormone levels will make you not want to eat anything.

Excessive hair growth on the face or other areas of the body that are typical of males is a common sign of a hormone imbalance in women. The condition is known as hirsutism, and it is often caused by an excess of androgen hormones such as testosterone.

WHAT IS HERBAL MEDICINE

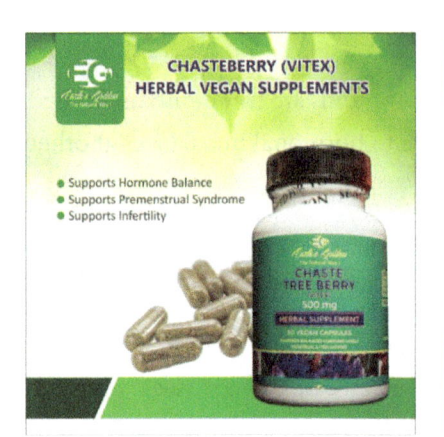

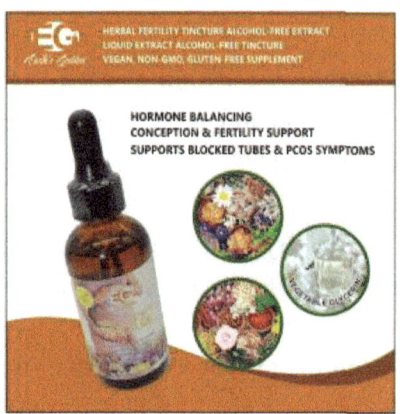

Herbal medicine, also known as herbalism or botanical medicine, is a traditional healing practice that involves using plants and their extracts for medicinal purposes. It is a holistic approach to healthcare that dates back thousands of years and is deeply rooted in various cultures and civilizations throughout history. It involves the use of parts of plants, such as leaves, roots, flowers, or bark, to create natural remedies that can help support the body's natural healing abilities.

The history of herbal medicine is vast and diverse, with evidence of its use dating back to ancient times. The knowledge of medicinal plants and their therapeutic properties has been passed down through generations, often through oral traditions and written texts.

One of the earliest known records of herbal medicine comes from ancient Mesopotamia (modern-day Iraq) around 3000 BCE. The

Sumerians, considered one of the oldest civilizations, documented their use of medicinal plants on clay tablets, including remedies for various ailments and diseases.

Ancient Egypt, renowned for its advanced medical practices, also embraced herbal medicine. The Ebers Papyrus, an Egyptian medical document dating back to around 1550 BCE, contains detailed information on the use of herbs for treating a wide range of conditions. The Egyptians recognized the healing properties of plants such as aloe vera, garlic, and frankincense.

In ancient Greece, herbal medicine flourished under the influence of notable figures such as Hippocrates and Dioscorides. Hippocrates, often called the "Father of Medicine," emphasized the importance of natural remedies and the body's innate ability to heal itself. His holistic approach to healthcare included the use of herbs and plant-based preparations.

Dioscorides, a Greek physician and pharmacologist, compiled a comprehensive herbal reference known as De Materia Medica in the 1st century C.E. This work documented over 600 medicinal plants and their therapeutic uses, serving as a valuable resource for herbalists throughout the ages.

Herbal medicine also thrived in ancient China, where it was an integral part of Traditional Chinese Medicine (T.C.M.). The Huangdi Neijing, also known as the Yellow Emperor's Inner Canon, is a seminal text that outlines the principles and practices of T.C.M. It includes extensive information on herbs to restore balance and promote health.

During the Middle Ages, herbal medicine continued to evolve in Europe. The works of herbalists like Hildegard of Bingen, a German abbess, and herbalist, contributed to the advancement of herbal knowledge. Her writings emphasized the comprehensive approach to healing and recognized the interconnectedness of the body, mind, and spirit.

In the Renaissance, herbal medicine experienced a resurgence, with notable figures such as Nicholas Culpeper making significant contributions. Culpeper's book, The English Physician, published in the 17th century, provided detailed information on herbal remedies accessible to the general population. His work helped democratize herbal medicine and empower individuals to control their health.

More recently, herbal medicine has seen a resurgence of interest and research. The founding father of modern herbal medicine is often attributed to the Austrian herbalist and physician Maria Treben. Her book, Health Through God's Pharmacy, published in 1980, popularized the use of herbs and their applications for various health conditions.

Today, herbal medicine continues to thrive as a complementary and alternative approach to healthcare. Scientific research and advancements in phytochemistry have provided valuable insights into the active constituents of plants and their mechanisms of action. Herbalists, naturopathic doctors, and other healthcare professionals integrate traditional wisdom with modern scientific knowledge to provide holistic and individualized treatment plans.

Herbal medicine holds immense potential for promoting health and well-being, offering natural alternatives, and supporting the body's innate healing abilities. As we delve deeper into the world of plants and their therapeutic properties, we uncover a rich tapestry of remedies that have been used for centuries, connecting us to our ancestral roots and a profound understanding of nature's healing power.

Herbal supplements are one of the most popular forms of herbal medicine. They are available in various forms, such as capsules, tablets, tinctures, powders, and teas. Herbal supplements contain active ingredients derived from plants believed to have therapeutic effects on the body.

Herbal supplements can be used for various health purposes, including improving digestion, reducing inflammation, boosting immune function, promoting sleep, managing stress and anxiety, and supporting healthy hormone balance.

When selecting herbal supplements, choosing products from reputable manufacturers that use high-quality, standardized extracts is important. Additionally, it is essential to read labels carefully, follow dosage instructions, and be aware of interactions with other medications.

Overall, incorporating herbal supplements into a healthy lifestyle can be a beneficial way to support overall health and well-being. However, it is vital to approach herbal supplements with caution and seek guidance from a qualified herbalist when necessary.

The use of herbs to treat hormone imbalances in women has a long history that dates to ancient times. Traditional healers and herbalists around the world have used different plants to alleviate various symptoms associated with hormone imbalances. For example, in traditional Chinese medicine, herbs such as Dong Quai, Ginger, and licorice root have been used for centuries to treat menstrual disorders, PMS, and other hormone-related conditions. Similarly, Ayurvedic medicine from India has used Ashwagandha, Shatavari, and other herbs to balance hormones and support reproductive health.

In the Western world, herbs such as Black cohosh, red clover, and Chaste berry have been used to relieve hot flashes, night sweats, and other menopausal symptoms. Additionally, herbs such as milk thistle and dandelion root have been used to support liver function, which can help to metabolize hormones more efficiently.

As modern science has progressed, research has confirmed the effectiveness of many of these traditional herbal remedies for hormone imbalances. Today, many women are turning to herbal remedies as a natural and safe alternative to conventional hormone replacement therapy.

Step into the enchanting world of herbal medicine as we journey through time and nature's bountiful remedies. This captivating book will delve into the secrets of hormonal balance and uncover the incredible power of herbal allies.

Our first stop is the mysterious Black Cohosh, an herb revered by Native American tribes for its ability to soothe menstrual discomfort and hormonal fluctuations. Through ancient legends and tales, we will unravel the history of this remarkable plant and explore its countless benefits. Join us as we uncover the wisdom of past generations and learn how Black Cohosh can guide your path to hormonal harmony.

Next, we will venture into Chinese medicine with Dong Quai, the beloved "female ginseng." Discover the captivating story behind this ancient herb, revered for centuries for its ability to nourish the blood and balance hormones. Let us unlock the secrets of Dong Quai's gentle strength as we explore its traditional uses and modern applications, empowering you to find balance and vitality.

As we journey further, we encounter the enchanting Chaste Tree Berry, also known as Vitex. Unveiling its rich history and folklore, we will uncover the secrets of this magical herb and its profound influence on hormonal health. Through fascinating case studies, you will witness the transformative power of Vitex and its role in harmonizing the intricate dance of hormones.

Prepare to be captivated by the ethereal beauty of Red Clover, a cherished herb revered for its abundance of nutrients and hormonal support. We will explore its storied past, from ancient civilizations to modern times, and unlock its extraordinary healing potential. Join us as we reveal the

NO MORE HORMONE IMBALANCES

captivating tales of Red Clover and discover how it can bring balance and radiance to your life.

Our journey takes a captivating turn as we delve into the world of Dog blood, a lesser-known herb with potent hormone-balancing properties. Immerse yourself in the folklore and traditions surrounding this remarkable plant and witness it's amazing effects through inspiring case studies. Discover the hidden wonders of Dog blood as we unlock its potential to restore equilibrium and vitality.

Elevate your senses and embrace the soothing touch of Evening Primrose, an exquisite flower that holds the secrets to hormonal wellness. As we uncover its historical significance and delve into its therapeutic benefits, you will witness the transformative power of Evening Primrose oil and its ability to relieve hormonal imbalances. Let its delicate fragrance and healing properties guide you towards balance and serenity.

Prepare to be captivated by the resilience and strength of Maca Root, an ancient herb revered by the indigenous people of the Andes. Through captivating tales and scientific insights, we will unravel the mysteries of Maca and its ability to nourish the endocrine system. Join us as we explore its adaptogenic qualities and discover how Maca can restore vitality and vitality to your hormonal journey.

The lush gardens of Red Raspberry leaf beckon us next, with their delicate leaves and remarkable healing properties. Embark on a botanical adventure as we uncover this cherished herb's historical uses and folklore. Witness the unique stories of women who have found solace and balance through Red Raspberry leaf and learn how it can support your hormonal health and overall well-being.

Our journey is only complete with the inclusion of Wild Yam, a plant revered for promoting hormonal balance and alleviating discomfort. Traverse the annals of time and uncover the historical significance of

Wild Yam as we unveil its therapeutic benefits and healing potential. Prepare to be inspired by the stories of women who have found solace in Wild Yam and embrace the transformation it can bring to your life.

Lastly, we invite you to unlock the hidden secrets of Burdock Root, a bonus herb with profound implications for hormonal health. Through captivating tales and traditional wisdom, we will reveal the remarkable qualities of this underground gem. Discover the healing powers of Burdock Root as we delve into its historical uses and explore its potential to cleanse, nourish, and restore harmony to your hormonal ecosystem.

With each turn of the page, you will be immersed in the rich tapestry of herbal medicine's history and its profound implications for hormonal health. From the ancient wisdom of indigenous cultures to today's innovative scientific research, this book will empower you with the knowledge and tools to embark on your transformative journey toward hormonal balance.

So, step into this world of botanical wonders, where ancient traditions and modern science intertwine, and let the healing power of nature guide you on the path to vibrant health and balanced hormones.

HERBS TO SUPPORT HORMONE IMBALANCES

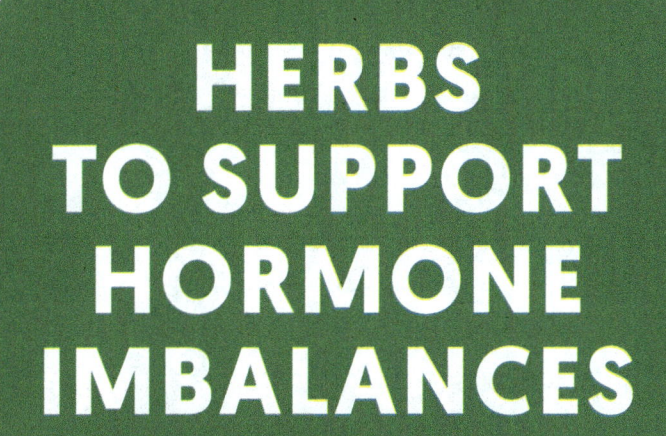

HERB 1
Black Cohosh Herb

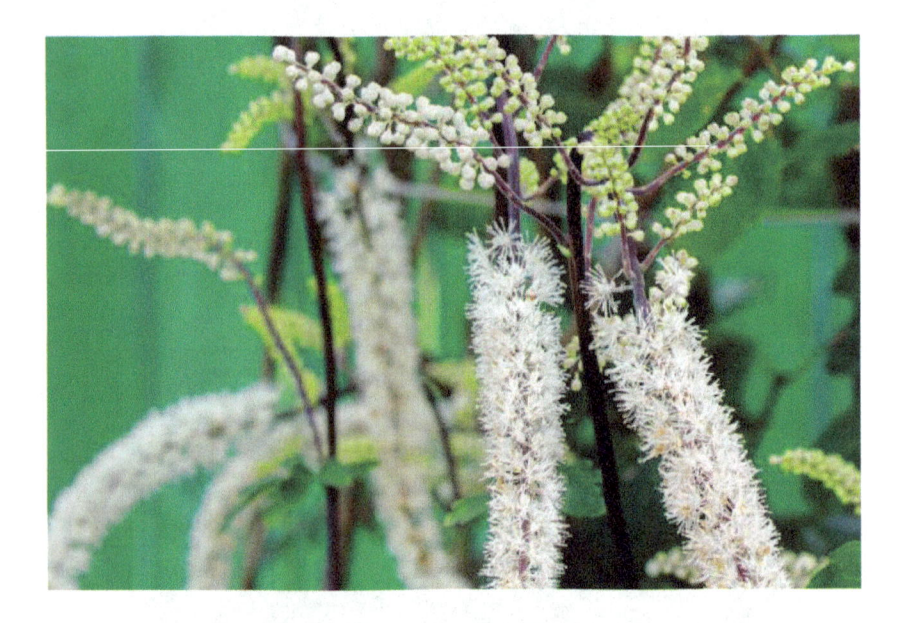

Imagine stepping into the enchanting depths of an ancient forest, where the secrets of nature's healing embrace you. In this mystical realm, we encounter a remarkable herb known as Black Cohosh, scientifically named Actaea Racemosa. Its name alone evokes a sense of mystery and intrigue, hinting at the profound wisdom it holds for our well-being.

Black Cohosh has a long and captivating history, deeply rooted in Native American traditions and folklore. For centuries, indigenous tribes revered this plant as a sacred ally, using it to address a variety of ailments and particularly valuing its ability to support women's health. The herb derived its name from the Algonquin language, where "cohosh" means "rough," alluding to the plant's gnarled appearance and the rough texture of its roots. The term "black" refers to the dark color of the source, which starkly contrasts with the vibrant green foliage above.

The Native American tribes of the eastern United States, such as the Cherokee and Iroquois, held Black Cohosh in high regard for its remarkable properties. They used it to remedy menstrual discomfort, menopausal symptoms, and various reproductive issues. The plant was often called "squawroot" or "women's root" due to its unique ability to support female reproductive health.

As European settlers arrived in North America, they began to recognize the incredible medicinal value of Black Cohosh. It was introduced to Europe in the mid-18th century, where it quickly gained popularity as a natural remedy. In traditional European herbal medicine, Black Cohosh alleviates menstrual cramps, regulates hormonal imbalances, and eases menopausal symptoms. Over time, a scientific exploration into the properties of Black Cohosh intensified, leading to numerous studies and clinical trials.

Researchers sought to unravel the mysteries behind this powerful herb and validate its traditional uses. While the exact mechanisms of Black Cohosh's actions are still being studied, it is believed to influence hormonal regulation, through its interactions with estrogen receptors.

Today, Black Cohosh remains a cherished herbal remedy for women's health concerns. It is widely used to alleviate menopausal symptoms such as hot flashes, mood swings, and sleep disturbances. Many women also turn to Black Cohosh for support during menstruation, finding relief from cramps, bloating, and hormonal fluctuations.

The deep-rooted history of Black Cohosh, intertwined with cultural traditions and scientific exploration, displays its enduring significance in herbal medicine. Its ability to support hormonal balance and relieve women's health concerns has made it a beloved herb worldwide.

As we continue our journey through herbal medicine, Black Cohosh will undoubtedly stand as a shining example of nature's wisdom and the profound impact it can have on our well-being. Let its story inspire you to embrace the healing power of plants and embark on a transformative journey toward hormonal harmony.

Case Studies on Black Cohosh

CASE STUDY #1

A study published in the Journal of Women's Health & Gender-Based Medicine followed 80 women experiencing menopausal symptoms who were given black cohosh extract twice daily for 12 weeks (about 3 months). The results showed a significant reduction in hot flashes, mood disturbances, and vaginal dryness, indicating an improvement in hormonal balance.

CASE STUDY #2

Another study published in the journal Maturitas involved 60 women with menopausal symptoms who were randomly assigned to receive either a black cohosh extract or a placebo for 12 weeks (about 3 months). The black cohosh group showed significant improvements in hot flashes, sweating, sleep disturbances, and vaginal dryness, indicating a positive effect on hormonal balance.

CASE STUDY #3

A case report published in the journal Menopause described a 53-year-old woman experiencing hot flashes, night sweats, and other menopausal symptoms. After taking black cohosh for six weeks, her symptoms improved significantly, and her hormone levels were found to be balanced.

CASE STUDY #4

In a case series published in the Journal of the American Board of Family Medicine, three women experiencing menopausal symptoms were given black cohosh extract, and all three reported improvements in their symptoms, including a reduction in hot flashes and improved sleep.

RECIPE 1

Black Cohosh Herbal Tea

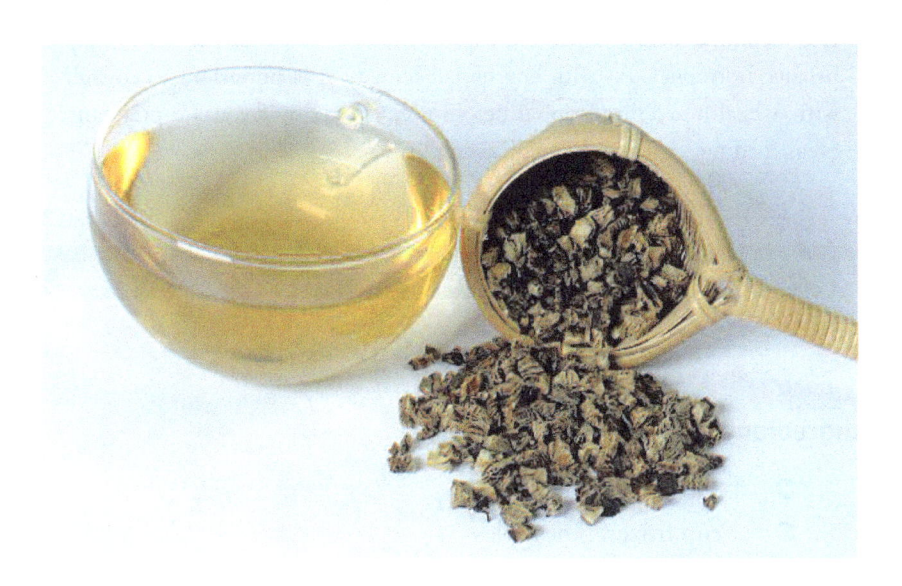

Ingredients:

- 1 tablespoon of dried Black Cohosh root
- 2 cups of water

Instructions:

Boil the water in a pot on the stove.

Add the dried Black Cohosh root to the pot of boiling water.

Reduce the heat to a simmer and let the mixture simmer for about 20 minutes.

Remove the pot from the heat and let it cool for a few minutes.

Strain the tea using a fine mesh strainer or cheesecloth.

Pour the tea into a mug and enjoy.

> Note: You can add a natural sweetener like agave, honey, or stevia if desired. It is recommended to drink 1-2 cups of Black Cohosh tea per day to help balance hormones. As with any herbal remedy, it is important to consult with a healthcare professional before use, especially if you are pregnant, breastfeeding, or have any medical conditions.

RECIPE 2

Black Cohosh Smoothie

Ingredients:

- 1 cup frozen dragon fruit
- 1 cup frozen pineapples
- 1/2 cup cashews
- 1/2 cup almond milk
- 1 tsp agave
- 1/2 tsp black cohosh powder

Instructions:

Add all ingredients to a blender and blend until smooth.

If the smoothie is too thick, add more almond milk as needed. Pour into a glass and enjoy!

RECIPE 3

Black Cohosh Juice

Ingredients:

- 2 Green apples
- 1 Cucumber
- 1 lemon
- 1 inch piece of ginger
- 2 large oranges
- 1/2 tsp black cohosh powder

Instructions:

Wash and chop the apples, orange, carrots, and ginger.

Juice the apples, carrots, orange, lemon, and ginger using a juicer.

Stir in the black cohosh root or powder until well combined.

Pour into a glass and enjoy!

HERB 2
Dong Quai Herb

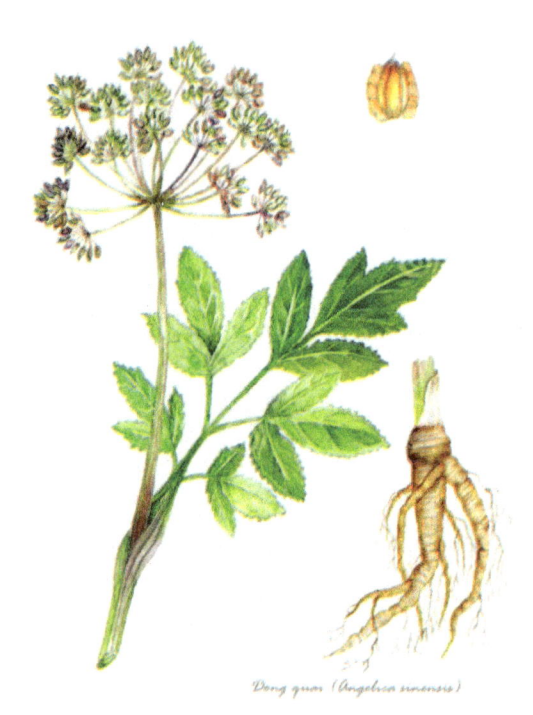

Dong quai (Angelica sinensis)

In herbal medicine, a magnificent plant known as Dong Quai exists, scientifically named Angelica sinensis. Like a graceful angelic presence, it has captivated the hearts and minds of healers and herbalists throughout history, offering profound benefits to those seeking balance and vitality.

Dong Quai is primarily grown in China, Korea, and Japan and is found in mountainous regions. It thrives in damp, shady areas and is typically harvested in the fall when the roots are the most potent. It belongs to the

Apiaceae family, which includes other plants such as celery, parsley, and carrots. It is also closely related to other medicinal herbs such as ginseng and licorice.

Dong Quai has a remarkable heritage deeply rooted in traditional Chinese medicine (T.C.M.). This herb has been revered and celebrated as an ideal female tonic for over two millennia. Its Chinese name, "Dang Gui," translates to "state of return," alluding to its ability to restore harmony and equilibrium to the body.

Legend has it that Dong Quai's discovery can be traced back to a Taoist monk named Qian Danou during the Tang Dynasty in ancient China. As the story goes, Qian Danou wandered through the mountains and came across a lush valley filled with aromatic herbs. Intrigued by their beauty, he began experimenting with their medicinal properties. It was during this exploration that he unearthed the remarkable qualities of Dong Quai, leading to its inclusion in the esteemed materia medica of T.C.M.

Dong Quai quickly became renowned for its affinity for women's health. It was considered an essential herb for supporting menstrual health, easing menstrual cramps, and promoting regularity. Additionally, it was believed to nourish and purify the blood, providing a gentle yet effective means to restore vitality and balance to the female reproductive system.

As knowledge of Dong Quai's benefits spread throughout China, its popularity grew, and it became a staple in T.C.M. formulations designed for women's wellness. Its traditional uses expanded to include support during menopause, postpartum recovery, and overall hormonal balance.

Over time, Dong Quai's reputation crossed borders and reached other parts of the world, captivating the interest of herbalists and holistic practitioners worldwide. Its recognition and use expanded beyond

T.C.M., gaining appreciation in Western herbal medicine for its potential therapeutic properties.

Modern scientific research has sought to explore the constituents and mechanisms behind Dong Quai's traditional uses. While our understanding continually evolves, studies have highlighted its potential as an antioxidant, anti-inflammatory, and hormone modulator. The herb is rich in bioactive compounds, including coumarins, phthalides, and polysaccharides, contributing to its diverse pharmacological effects.

Today, Dong Quai is widely embraced as a botanical ally for women's health and hormonal balance. It is commonly used to alleviate menstrual discomfort, support fertility, and address symptoms associated with menopause. Additionally, it is renowned for its ability to nourish and purify the blood, promoting overall vitality and well-being.

The centuries-old legacy of Dong Quai within the realm of herbal medicine is a testament to its profound impact on women's health. Its rich history, deeply intertwined with traditional Chinese medicine, highlights its enduring significance and popularity as a beloved herb.

As we embark on our journey through the world of herbal medicine, let the story of Dong Quai inspire us to honor the ancient wisdom of plants and embrace their transformative potential. May Dong Quai's gentle yet powerful presence guides us toward harmony, vitality, and optimal well- being.

Case Studies on Dong Quai

CASE STUDY #1: MENOPAUSAL SYMPTOMS

A 52-year-old woman was experiencing severe hot flashes, night sweats, and mood swings associated with menopause. She had been experiencing these symptoms for over a year and had tried several over-the-counter remedies with little success.

She decided to try Dong Quai, which she had read about in a natural health magazine. She took 500mg (about half the weight of a small paper clip) of Dong Quai twice a day for two weeks and reported a significant improvement in her symptoms. Her hot flashes and night sweat decreased, and her mood swings became less severe.

After one month of taking Dong Quai, she reported feeling like her old self again. Her energy levels increased, and she felt more in control of her emotions.

CASE STUDY #2: DYSMENORRHEA

A 24-year-old woman was experiencing severe menstrual cramps and bloating associated with her period. She had been taking over-the-counter pain relievers, but they provided little relief.

She consulted with a traditional Chinese medicine practitioner, who recommended Dong Quai. She took 1000mg (about the weight of a small paper clip) of Dong Quai daily for two weeks leading up to her period.

During her next menstrual cycle, she reported a significant reduction in her cramps and bloating. She was able to go about her daily activities without feeling overwhelmed by pain and discomfort.

After several months of taking Dong Quai, she reported that her menstrual symptoms had improved significantly, and she was able to manage them without relying on over-the-counter medications.

APRIL HEATH-WHITE, M.S., B.S., A.A.

RECIPE 1

Dong Quai Herbal Tea

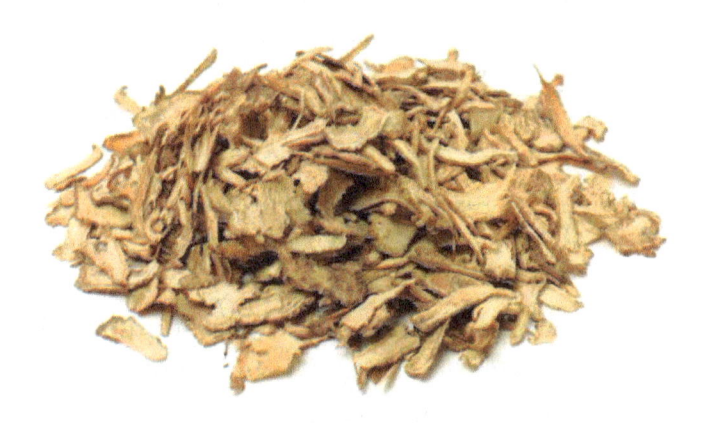

Ingredients:

- 1-2 teaspoons of dried Dong Quai root
- 1 cup of water
- agave (optional)

Instructions:

Add the dried Dong Quai root to a teapot or infuser.

Heat water until it comes to a boil, then pour it over the Dong Quai root in the teapot or infuser.

Let the tea steep for 5-10 minutes.

Strain the tea into a cup.

Add agave to taste, if desired.

Enjoy your Dong Quai herbal tea!

Note: Dong Quai is considered safe when consumed in moderation. However, it is important to consult with a healthcare professional before using it, especially if you are pregnant or breastfeeding, have a history of blood clots, or are taking any medications that may interact with Dong Quai.

RECIPE 2

Dong Quai Smoothie

Ingredients:

- 1 banana
- 1 cup frozen berries (such as blueberries or strawberries)
- 1/2 cup plain Greek yogurt
- 1/2 cup almond milk
- 1 tsp agave
- 1 tsp dried Dong Quai root

Instructions:

Add all ingredients to a blender and blend until smooth.

If the smoothie is too thick, add more almond milk as needed.

Pour into a glass and enjoy your Dong Quai smoothie!

APRIL HEATH-WHITE, M.S., B.S., A.A.

RECIPE 3

Dong Quai Juice

Ingredients:

- 2 large apples
- 2 medium carrots
- 1 inch piece of ginger
- 1/2 lemon
- 1 tsp dried Dong Quai root

Instructions:

Wash and chop the apples, carrots, and ginger.

Juice the apples, carrots, ginger, and lemon using a juicer.

Stir in the dried Dong Quai root until well combined.

Pour into a glass and enjoy your Dong Quai juice!

▶ HERB 3
Chaste Tree Berry (Vitex) Herb

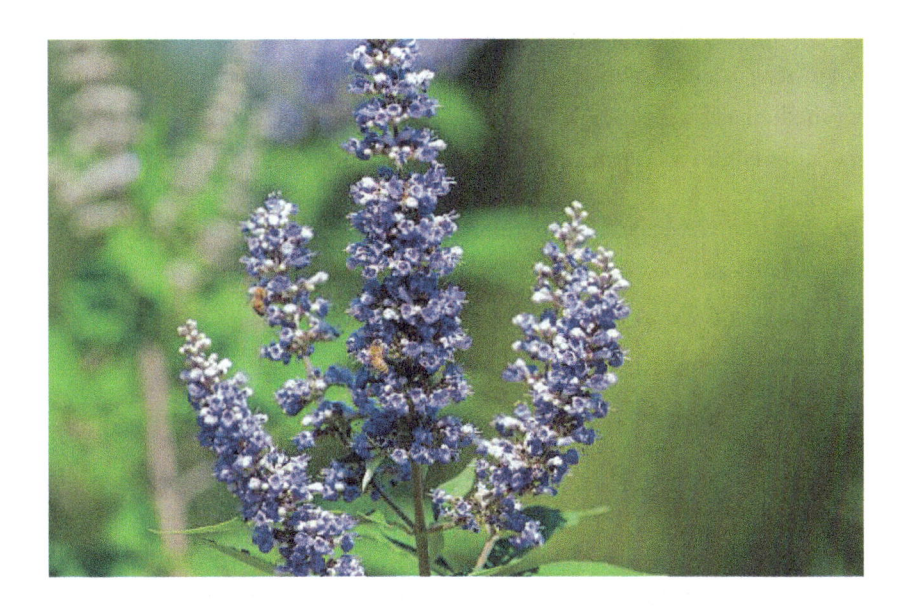

At the heart of herbal medicine stands a remarkable plant known as the Chaste tree, scientifically called Vitex agnus-castus. This extraordinary herb has a history deeply rooted in ancient civilizations, captivating the attention of herbalists and healers for centuries with its profound effects on women's health.

Vitex is native to the Mediterranean region but is now widely grown in many parts of the world, including Europe, Asia, Africa, and North America. It thrives in warm, sunny climates and is typically found in dry, rocky areas. It belongs to the Lamiaceae family, which includes other plants such as mint, basil, and sage. It is closely related to medicinal herbs, such as rosemary and lavender.

Chaste tree berry derives its name from its traditional use as an herb to help monks maintain celibacy. In ancient times, it was believed that chewing the berries of this tree could suppress sexual desire, hence earning it the moniker "Chaste." However, it is essential to note that the herb does not possess actual contraceptive properties.

This illustrious herb originates in the Mediterranean, thriving in warm and sunny climates. It has been cherished since the days of ancient Greece when it was first described by the renowned physician Hippocrates for its medicinal qualities. Theophrastus, a student of Aristotle, also noted its benefits and recommended it for various female ailments.

The chaste tree belongs to the Verbenaceae family, which includes plants with aromatic properties and delicate flowers. The Chaste tree is a powerful medicinal herb within this family, specifically revered for its influence on hormone balance.

Throughout history, the Chaste tree has been celebrated for its ability to support women's reproductive health. Traditional herbalists used it to address many menstrual issues, including irregular cycles, premenstrual syndrome (P.M.S.), and hormonal imbalances. The berries of the Chaste tree were commonly prepared as an herbal infusion or tincture, and the resulting preparation was administered to help bring balance to the female reproductive system.

The herb's popularity and recognition spread beyond the Mediterranean, finding its way into other traditional systems of medicine. It became a significant component in Ayurvedic medicine, known as "Nirgundi." In this ancient Indian system, the Chaste tree addressed female reproductive disorders, enhanced fertility, and supported overall hormonal balance.

Modern scientific research has sought to uncover the mechanisms behind the Chaste tree's traditional uses. The herb has been found to exert its effects on the pituitary gland, which plays a crucial role in regulating hormone production. The active compounds in the Chaste tree, including flavonoids and essential oils, act on the pituitary gland, promoting the production of luteinizing hormone (L.H.) and suppressing the secretion of follicle-stimulating hormone (F.S.H.). This hormonal balance can contribute to normalizing the menstrual cycle and reducing symptoms associated with hormonal imbalances.

The extensive historical use and scientific interest in the Chaste tree have established it as a valuable botanical ally for women's health. It is widely recognized as a natural remedy to help regulate menstrual cycles, alleviate P.M.S. symptoms, and support fertility. It is particularly favored by those seeking a gentle and integrated approach to hormonal balance.

As we embrace the wisdom of the Chaste tree and delve into the world of herbal medicine, let us honor the knowledge passed down through generations. May the story of the Chaste tree inspire us to nurture our bodies, celebrate the delicate dance of hormones, and embrace the power of nature's remedies in our pursuit of optimal well-being.

Case Studies on Chaste Tree Berry (Vitex)

CASE STUDY #1:
PREMENSTRUAL SYNDROME (PMS)

A 35-year-old woman was experiencing severe PMS symptoms, including bloating, breast tenderness, and mood swings, for several months. She had tried several over-the-counter remedies, but they provided little relief.

She consulted with a naturopathic doctor, who recommended Chaste tree berry. She took 500mg (about half the weight of a small paper clip) of Chaste tree berry extract daily for three months.

After three months of taking Chaste tree berry, she reported a significant reduction in her PMS symptoms. Her bloating and breast tenderness decreased, and her mood swings became less severe.

CASE STUDY #2: INFERTILITY

A 32-year-old woman had been trying to conceive for over a year without success. She had been diagnosed with polycystic ovary syndrome (PCOS) and was experiencing irregular menstrual cycles and hormonal imbalances.

She consulted with a fertility specialist, who recommended Chaste tree berry. She took 500mg (about half the weight of a small paper clip) of Chaste tree berry extract daily for six months.

After six months of taking Chaste tree berry, she reported a significant improvement in her menstrual cycles and hormonal imbalances. She also became pregnant shortly after completing the six-month treatment.

RECIPE 1

Chaste Tree Berry Smoothie

Ingredients:

- 1 banana
- 1 cup frozen mixed berries
- 1/2 cup almond butter
- 1/2 cup almond milk
- 1 tsp honey
- 1 tsp Chaste tree berry extract

Instructions:

Add all ingredients to a blender and blend until smooth.

If the smoothie is too thick, add more almond milk as needed.

Pour into a glass and enjoy your Chaste tree berry smoothie!

RECIPE 2

Chaste Tree Berry Juice

Ingredients:

- 1 large Watermelon
- 1 large cucumber
- 1 inch piece of mint
- 1 inch piece of basil
- 1 tsp Chaste tree berry extract

Instructions:

Wash and chop the watermelon, cucumber, mint, and basil.

Juice the watermelon, cucumber, mint, and basil using a juicer.

Stir in the Chaste tree berry extract until well combined.

Pour into a glass and enjoy your Chaste tree berry juice!

RECIPE 3

Chaste Tree Berry Herbal Tea

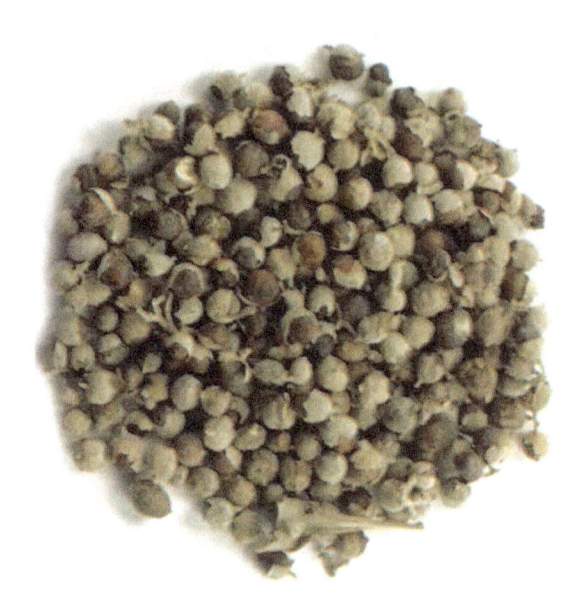

Ingredients:

- 1 tsp dried Chaste tree berries
- 1 cup water
- Honey (optional)

Instructions:

Add the dried Chaste tree berries to a teapot or infuser.

Heat water until it comes to a boil, then pour it over the Chaste tree berries in the teapot or infuser.

Let the tea steep for 5-10 minutes. Strain the tea into a cup.

Add honey to taste, if desired.

Enjoy your Chaste tree berry herbal tea!

> Note: It is important to speak with your doctor or a qualified healthcare practitioner before using Chaste tree berry, as it may interact with certain medications. Additionally, the taste of Chaste tree berry can be quite strong and bitter, so you may need to adjust the amount of Chaste tree berry to suit your taste preferences.

HERB 4
Red Clover Herb

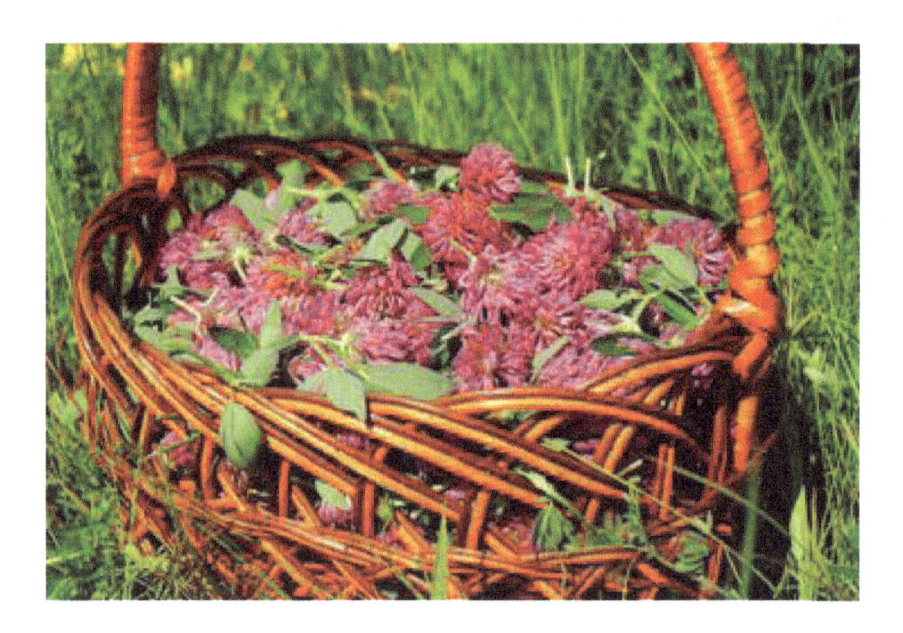

Deep in the meadows and fields, a vibrant and enchanting herb known as Red Clover, scientifically named Trifolium pratense, graces the landscape with its delicate blooms. With a history spanning centuries, this remarkable plant has captured the attention of herbalists and natural healers worldwide.

Belonging to the legume family, Fabaceae, Red Clover is a perennial herbaceous plant characterized by its vibrant red flowers, which stand proudly on slender stems. It is native to Europe, Asia, and North Africa but has since found its way to various regions across the globe due to its medicinal properties.

Red Clover is known for its versatility and therapeutic potential throughout history. Its use traces back to ancient civilizations, where it is revered for its ability to support various aspects of health. In traditional herbal practices, it is used as a blood purifier, an expectorant, and a remedy for skin conditions.

Red Clover's popularity as a women's herb also dates back centuries. It recognized for its potential to support hormonal balance and relieve symptoms associated with menopause and premenstrual discomfort. The herb's affinity for female health led to its widespread use in traditional systems of medicine, including Traditional Chinese Medicine and Ayurveda.

In Traditional Chinese Medicine, Red Clover is called "Ting Hsien" and regarded for its cooling properties. It is believed to clear heat and toxins from the body and promote detoxification.

Similarly, in Ayurveda, Red Clover is known as "Punarvana" or "Shveta Parpati" and is used to support reproductive health and address imbalances related to menstruation and menopause.

The rich legacy of Red Clover also extends to Western herbal traditions. During the 19th century, it gained significant recognition as a key ingredient in various herbal formulations. It is a gentle and supportive remedy for menopausal symptoms, including hot flashes, night sweats, and mood swings. Red Clover's reputation as a women's herb spread rapidly, solidifying its place in herbal medicine practices across the globe.

Modern scientific research has shed light on the potential mechanisms behind Red Clover's therapeutic effects. The herb contains various compounds, including isoflavones, flavonoids, and phytoestrogens, which have estrogenic activity. These plant-based compounds believed to interact with estrogen receptors in the body, supporting hormonal balance.

Today, Red Clover continues to be embraced by herbalists and health enthusiasts alike. It is often used as an ingredient in herbal teas, tinctures, and supplements, offering a natural approach to promoting women's health and well-being.

As we delve into the realm of herbal medicine and the captivating story of Red Clover, let us honor the ancient wisdom passed down through generations. May the legacy of this vibrant herb inspire us to seek harmony within our bodies, embrace the healing power of nature, and embark on a holistic wellness journey.

Case Studies on Red Clover

CASE STUDY #1

A 48-year-old woman with hot flashes and night sweats was given a red clover supplement containing 40 mg (about half the weight of a business card) of isoflavones per day. After 12 weeks (about 3 months) of treatment, the woman reported a significant reduction in hot flashes and night sweats, as well as an improvement in her overall quality of life.

CASE STUDY #2

A 45-year-old woman with irregular menstrual cycles and premenstrual symptoms was given a red clover supplement containing 80 mg (about the weight of a business card) of isoflavones per day. After three months of treatment, the woman reported a significant reduction in premenstrual symptoms, as well as an improvement in the regularity of her menstrual cycles.

CASE STUDY #3

A 50-year-old woman with vaginal dryness and low libido was given a red clover supplement containing 80 mg (about the weight of a business card) of isoflavones per day. After eight weeks of treatment, the woman reported an improvement in vaginal lubrication and an increase in libido.

RECIPE 1

Red Clover Smoothie

Ingredients:

- 1 cup fresh or frozen Papaya
- 1/2 cup cold pressed apple juice
- 1/2 cup frozen pineapples
- 1 cup of ice
- 1/2 cup of mangoes
- 1 tsp red clover blossoms (dried or fresh)

Instructions:

In a blender, combine all the fruits

Add the red clover blossoms to the blender.

Blend all ingredients together until smooth and well combined.

If the mixture is too thick, add more apple until it reaches your desired consistency.

Pour the smoothie into a glass and enjoy immediately.

Optional: You can also add a scoop of protein powder or a handful of spinach for extra nutrients.

Blend all ingredients in a blender until smooth. Enjoy!

RECIPE 2

Red Clover Juice

Ingredients:

- 2 cups of fresh red clover flowers
- 1 piece of mint
- 1 inch piece of fresh basil
- 1 Watermelon

Instructions:

Rinse the red clover flowers in chilly water and remove any dirt or debris.

Wash basil and mint.

Wash the watermelon and then chop it into smaller pieces.

Add all the ingredients into a blender or juicer and blend until smooth.

Pour the juice into a glass and serve immediately.

Optional: You can strain the juice through a fine mesh strainer or cheesecloth to remove any pulp, but it is not necessary. You can also add honey or another natural sweetener to taste.

RECIPE 3

Red Clover Herbal Tea

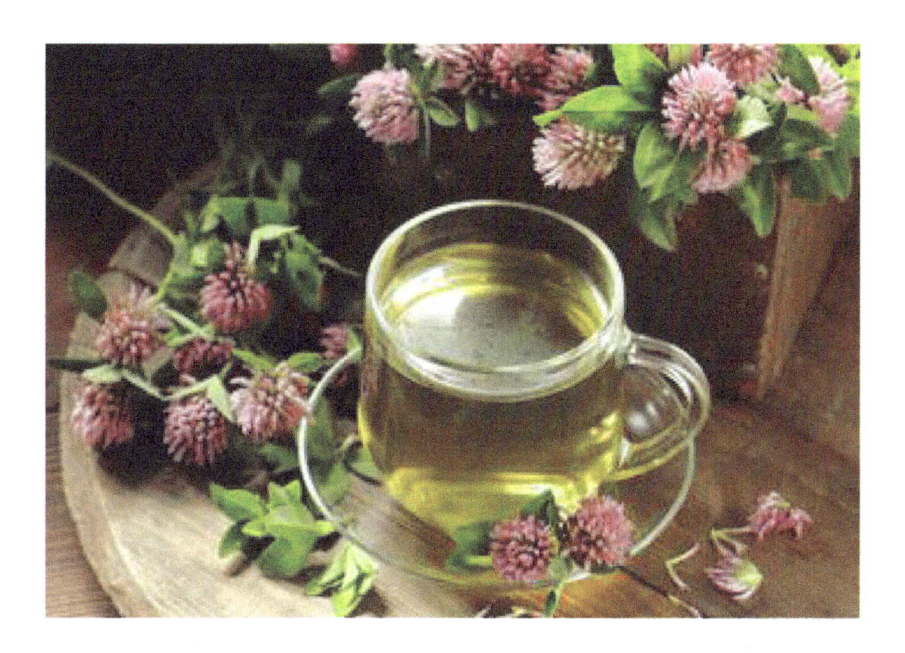

Ingredients:

- 1 tablespoon dried red clover blossoms
- 1 cup water
- Honey or lemon (optional)

Instructions:

Boil 1 cup of water in a saucepan or kettle.

Add 1 tablespoon of dried red clover blossoms to the hot water.

Cover the saucepan with a lid and let the tea steep for 10-15 minutes.

Strain the tea through a fine mesh strainer or cheesecloth.

Add honey or lemon, if desired, for additional flavor.

Serve the tea hot or cold.

> Note: Red clover tea can be consumed 1-3 times daily. It is recommended to start with a small amount and gradually increase the dose. It is also important to talk to a healthcare provider before using red clover, especially if taking medication or having a medical condition.

HERB 5

Sanguisorba Officinalis (Dog Blood) Herb

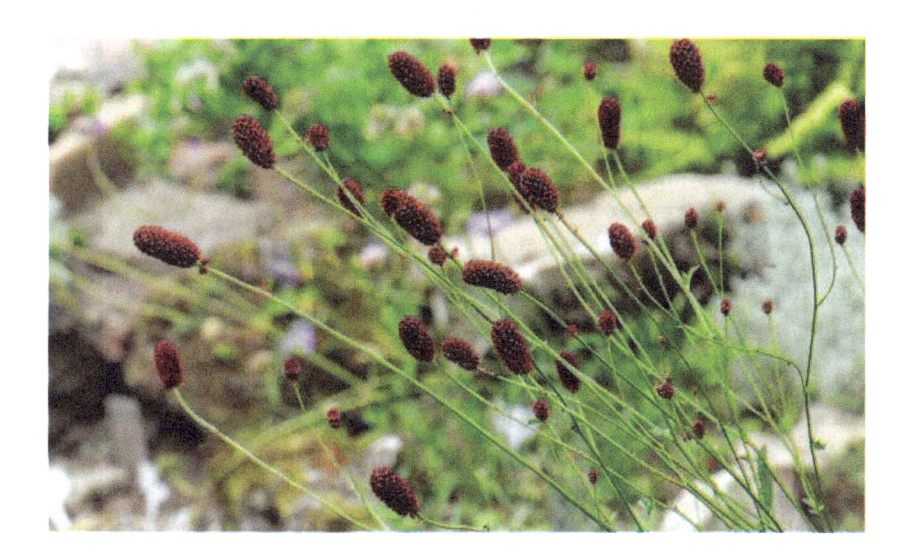

Deep within herbal medicine is a remarkable herb with a captivating name - Dog Blood Herb, scientifically known as Sanguisorba officinalis. This unique herb has a rich history that stretches back through the ages, captivating the attention of herbalists and healers across diverse cultures and continents.

Belonging to the family Rosaceae, Dog Blood Herb is a perennial flowering plant characterized by its elegant and graceful appearance. Its botanical name, Sanguisorba, derives from the Latin words "sanguis," meaning blood, and "sorbeo," meaning to absorb, alluding to the herb's historical association with blood-related conditions and its reputed ability to promote healthy blood flow.

Dog Blood Herb's origins can be traced to various regions, including Europe, Asia, and North America. It is native to these areas, has been cultivated, and used medicinally by distinct cultures throughout history. Its striking appearance, with feathery leaves and unusual cylindrical flower spikes, made it a notable plant in traditional herbal practices.

Throughout ancient times, Dog Blood Herb earned a reputation as a potent medicinal plant. In traditional Chinese medicine, it is referred to as "Di Yu" or "Xian He Cao." It has been used for centuries to promote blood circulation, alleviate bleeding disorders, and support overall health and vitality. Its use in Chinese herbal formulas is attributed to its astringent and hemostatic properties, which are valued for their ability to staunch bleeding and promote wound healing.

In European herbal traditions, Dog Blood Herb is regarded for its potential to address various health concerns. It is often employed as a medicinal tonic for its ability to support digestive health, relieve diarrhea, and regulate menstrual bleeding. Its astringent properties are believed to strengthen and tone tissues, making it a valuable remedy for conditions characterized by excessive bleeding or fluid loss.

Dog Blood Herb's historical association with blood-related conditions and its use as a hemostatic agent also made it a popular remedy for treating hemorrhoids, nosebleeds, and other bleeding disorders. Its ability to constrict blood vessels and reduce bleeding led to its inclusion in herbal formulas and remedies designed to address these ailments.

As we explore the fascinating history of Dog Blood Herb, we witness the legacy of this unique botanical unfolding. From ancient Chinese medicine to traditional European herbal practices, its reputation as a valuable therapeutic herb has stood the test of time.

Today, Dog Blood Herb continues to be celebrated in herbal medicine circles for its potential health benefits. It is used in various forms, including teas, tinctures, and topical applications, offering a natural approach to support healthy blood circulation, relieve bleeding disorders, and promote overall well-being.

Let the story of Dog Blood Herb inspire us to appreciate the intricate wisdom of nature and the profound healing potential found within its abundant offerings. Its historical significance reminds us of the powerful constructive interaction between humans and the plant kingdom as we continue our journey towards optimal health and vitality.

Case Studies on Sanguisorba Officinalis (Dog Blood) Herb

CASE STUDIES # 1

A study published in the journal Integrative Cancer Therapies followed 32 breast cancer patients who were undergoing chemotherapy. Half of the patients were given a combination of Sanguisorba officinalis and other herbal extracts, while the other half were given a placebo. The group taking the herbal extracts reported fewer side effects from chemotherapy, such as fatigue and nausea.

CASE STUDIES # 2

In another study published in the journal Phytomedicine, 60 women with menopausal symptoms were given either a Sanguisorba officinalis extract or a placebo. The group taking the extract reported significant improvements in symptoms such as hot flashes and night sweats.

CASE STUDIES # 3

A case study published in the Journal of Alternative and Complementary Medicine followed a woman with endometriosis, a condition where tissue like the lining of the uterus grows outside of it, causing pain and other symptoms. The woman took a combination of Sanguisorba officinalis and other herbal extracts and reported a significant reduction in pain and other symptoms.

CASE STUDIES # 4

In a study published in the Journal of Ethnopharmacology, Sanguisorba officinalis was shown to have anti-inflammatory effects in mice. The researchers concluded that the herb may be useful in treating inflammatory diseases in humans.

RECIPE 1

Sanguisorba Officinalis Smoothie

Ingredients:

- 1 cup frozen mangoes, Pineapples, Strawberries
- 1 cup of Coconut water
- 1 tablespoon honey
- 1 teaspoon Sanguisorba Officinalis powder (or finely chopped fresh herb)

Instructions:

Combine all ingredients in a blender and blend until smooth.

If the smoothie is too thick, add additional coconut water until desired consistency is reached.

Pour into a glass and enjoy.

Note: Sanguisorba Officinalis is a potent herb and should be used with caution.

RECIPE 2

Sanguisorba Officinalis Juice

Ingredients:

- 1/2 cup fresh Sanguisorba Officinalis leaves and stems
- 1 Pineapple
- 1 cucumber
- 1 lemon
- 1 inch ginger

Instructions:

Wash and chop the Sanguisorba Officinalis leaves and stems.

Cut the pineapple, cucumber, and lemon into chunks.

Peel and grate the ginger.

Add all the ingredients to a juicer and extract the juice.

Pour the juice into a glass and serve immediately.

Note: If you do not have a juicer, you can blend the ingredients in a blender and then strain the juice using a fine-mesh sieve or cheesecloth.

APRIL HEATH-WHITE, M.S., B.S., A.A.

RECIPE 3

Sanguisorba Officinalis Herbal Tea

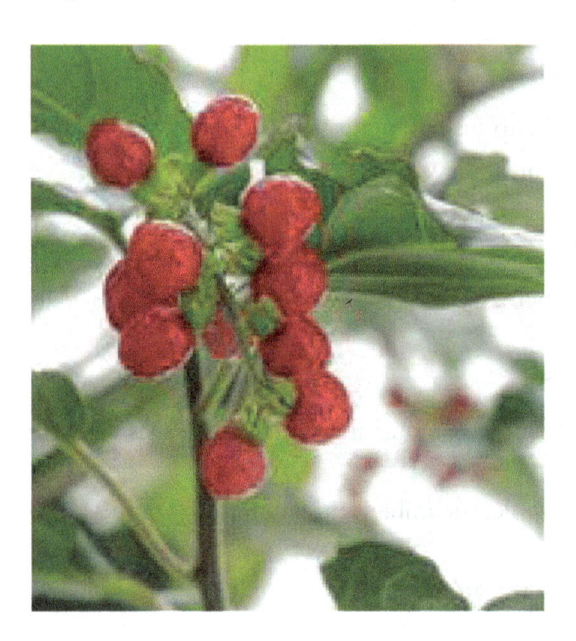

Ingredients:

- 1 tablespoon dried Sanguisorba Officinalis root
- 2 cups of water
- Honey (optional)

Instructions:

Bring 2 cups of water to a boil in a small pot.

Add 1 tablespoon of dried Sanguisorba Officinalis root to the boiling water.

Reduce the heat and let the mixture simmer for 10-15 minutes.

Strain the tea using a fine mesh strainer or cheesecloth.

Add honey to taste, if desired.

Enjoy your Sanguisorba Officinalis herbal tea hot or cold.

Note: It is important to consult with a healthcare professional before incorporating Sanguisorba Officinalis or any other herbal remedies into your diet, especially if you have any underlying health conditions or are taking medication.

HERB 6

Evening Primrose Herb

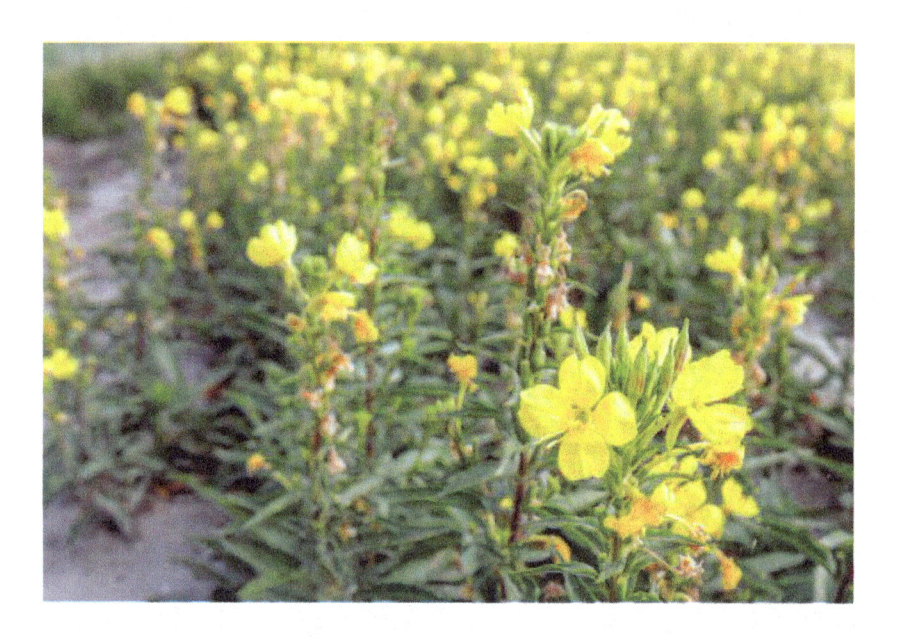

Step into the world of botanical wonders, where the enchanting Evening Primrose plant takes center stage. Known by its scientific name Oenothera biennis, this remarkable herb has a fascinating history deeply intertwined with human civilization and the pursuit of wellness.

Belonging to the Onagraceae family, the Evening Primrose plant displays its vibrant yellow flowers, which bloom in the Evening and give off a sweet, delicate fragrance. Native to North America, this perennial plant has also found a home in other regions across the globe due to its captivating beauty and medicinal potential.

The history of the Evening Primrose plant stretches back centuries, with Indigenous tribes in North America utilizing its various parts for medicinal and culinary purposes. These wise cultures recognized the plant's valuable properties and employed it in herbal remedies to address multiple ailments.

During the 17th and 18th centuries, European explorers and botanists encountered the Evening Primrose plant during their journeys to the New World. They were captivated by its striking appearance and intrigued by the potential medicinal benefits hidden within its seeds, leaves, and roots.

Since then, the Evening Primrose plant has been extensively studied and cultivated for its valuable oil extracted from its seeds. The oil, commonly called Evening Primrose oil, has gained widespread popularity as a dietary supplement and topical treatment due to its high content of essential fatty acids, especially gamma-linolenic acid (G.L.A.).

Evening Primrose oil has been used for various purposes, focusing on women's health. Many have embraced it as a natural remedy to support hormonal balance and alleviate symptoms associated with menstrual discomfort, premenstrual syndrome (P.M.S.), and menopause. Its potential anti-inflammatory properties have also made it a sought-after option for managing skin conditions such as eczema and acne.

The Evening Primrose plant's deep-rooted connection with human health continues to captivate herbal enthusiasts, researchers, and health practitioners. Through careful cultivation and extraction methods, the plant's beneficial properties have been harnessed and made accessible to individuals seeking natural alternatives for wellness.

As we delve into the story of the Evening Primrose plant, we unveil its remarkable journey from ancient healing traditions to modern-day applications. Its presence in gardens, herbal medicine cabinets, and cosmetic formulations is a testament to its enduring significance in our quest for vitality and well-being.

Embrace the allure of Evening Primrose and its golden blooms as you explore the rich tapestry of its history, medicinal benefits, and rightful place among nature's extraordinary botanical treasures.

Case Studies on Evening Primrose

CASE STUDY #1

A study published in the Journal of the American Academy of Dermatology in 2013 evaluated the use of evening primrose oil in the treatment of atopic dermatitis. The study involved 30 participants randomly assigned to receive evening primrose oil or a placebo for 12 weeks (about 3 months). The results showed that the group receiving evening primrose oil had a significant improvement in symptoms, including itching and redness, compared to the placebo group.

CASE STUDY #2

Another study published in the Journal of Rheumatology in 2000 evaluated the use of evening primrose oil in the treatment of rheumatoid arthritis. The study involved 49 randomly assigned participants to receive evening primrose oil or a placebo for 6 months. The results showed that the group receiving evening primrose oil had a significant reduction in joint pain and stiffness compared to the placebo group.

CASE STUDY #3

A case report published in the Journal of Obstetrics and Gynaecology in 2012 described the use of evening primrose oil in the treatment of breast pain associated with fibrocystic breast disease. The report described a patient who had been experiencing breast pain for several years and had not responded to other treatments. The patient began taking evening primrose oil and reported a significant improvement in symptoms after just one month of treatment.

CASE STUDY #4

A study published in the International Journal of Obesity in 2014 evaluated the use of evening primrose oil in the treatment of obesity-related inflammation. The study involved 30 participants randomly assigned to receive evening primrose oil or a placebo for 12 weeks (about 3 months). The results showed that the group receiving evening primrose oil had a significant reduction in inflammatory markers compared to the placebo group.

RECIPE 1

Evening Primrose Herbal Tea

Ingredients:

- 1-2 teaspoons of dried evening primrose leaves or flowers
- 1 cup of hot water
- Optional: honey or lemon for flavor

Instructions:

Place the evening primrose leaves or flowers into a tea infuser or strainer.

Pour hot water over the tea infuser/strainer and let it steep for 5-10 minutes.

Remove the tea infuser/strainer and discard the used leaves/flowers.

Add honey or lemon to taste (optional).

Enjoy your evening primrose herbal tea!

> Note: It is important to use high-quality dried evening primrose leaves or flowers for the best flavor and health benefits. If you are pregnant or breastfeeding, have a bleeding disorder, or take blood-thinning medications, it is important to talk to your healthcare provider before consuming evening primrose tea or any other supplements.

RECIPE 2

Evening Primrose Smoothie with Pineapple, Mango, and Coconut Water

Ingredients:

- 1 cup frozen pineapple chunks
- 1 cup frozen mango chunks
- 1 tablespoon Evening Primrose oil
- 1 cup coconut water
- Optional: sweetener of your choice (such as honey or agave)

Instructions:

Add the frozen pineapple and mango chunks to a blender.

Add the Evening Primrose oil and coconut water.

Blend on high until smooth and creamy.

Taste and add sweetener if desired.

Pour into a glass and enjoy your delicious and healthy Evening Primrose smoothie!

RECIPE 3

Strawberry Evening Primrose Smoothie

Ingredients:

- 1 cup frozen strawberries
- 1 banana
- 1 tablespoon Evening Primrose oil
- 1 cup almond milk
- Optional: sweetener of your choice (such as honey or agave)

Instructions:

Add the frozen strawberries and banana to a blender.

Add the Evening Primrose oil and almond milk.

Blend on high until smooth and creamy.

Taste and add sweetener if desired.

Pour into a glass and enjoy your refreshing and healthy Strawberry Evening Primrose smoothie!

APRIL HEATH-WHITE, M.S., B.S., A.A.

RECIPE 4

Evening Primrose juice with kale, spinach, cucumber, green apples, and ginger

Ingredients:

- 1 cup kale leaves
- 1 cup spinach leaves
- 1 cucumber, chopped
- 2 green apples, chopped
- 1-inch piece of ginger, peeled and grated
- 1 tablespoon Evening Primrose oil
- 1/2 cup water

Instructions:

Add the kale, spinach, cucumber, green apples, and ginger to a juicer.

Juice the ingredients until smooth.

Pour the juice into a blender.

Add the Evening Primrose oil and water to the blender.

Blend on high until smooth and creamy.

Pour the juice into a glass and enjoy your healthy and refreshing Evening Primrose juice!

> Note: You can adjust the ingredients to your liking and add more water if you prefer a thinner consistency. Also, be sure to use high-quality Evening Primrose oil for the best flavor and health benefits.

HERB 7
Maca Root Herb

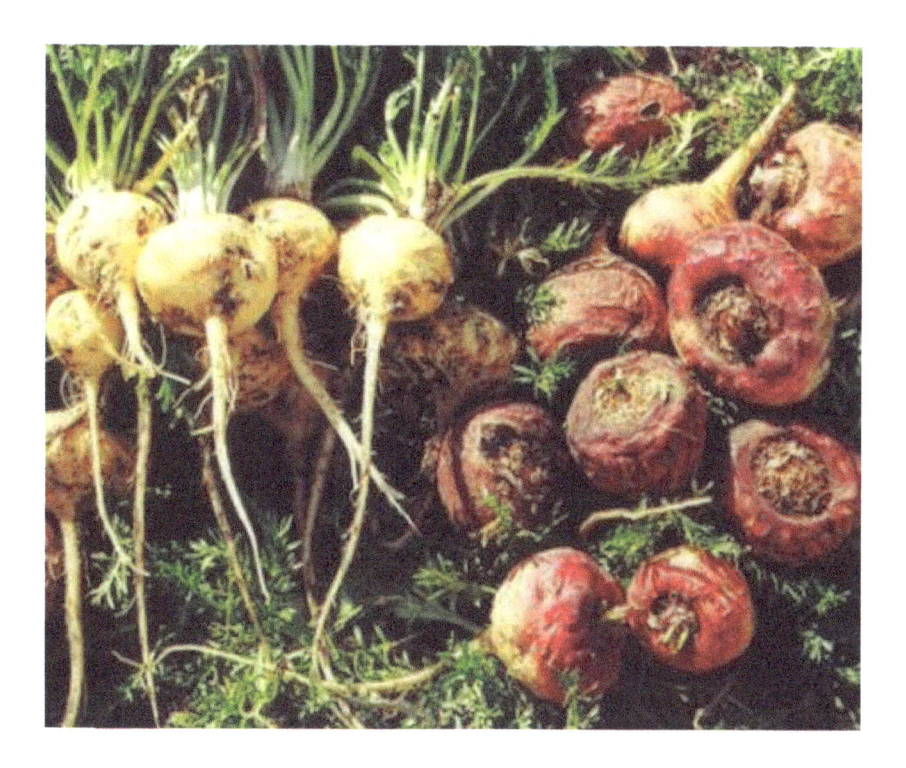

Maca root, scientifically known as Lepidium meyenii, is an herbaceous plant native to Peru's high-altitude regions of the Andes Mountains. It belongs to the Brassicaceae family, which includes other well-known plants like broccoli, cabbage, and radish.

The history of maca root dates back thousands of years, as it has been cultivated and used by the indigenous people of the Andes for its medicinal properties. It holds significant cultural and traditional value in Peru, where it has been a staple in their diet and herbal medicine practices.

Maca root was highly revered by the ancient Incas, who considered it a valuable and sacred plant. It was believed to enhance energy, stamina, and fertility and was often consumed by warriors before battles. The root was also known for improving mood, enhancing libido, and promoting overall well-being.

Traditionally, maca root was sun-dried and consumed raw or cooked. It was used to make porridge, beverages, and various culinary preparations. Over time, its popularity has spread globally, and it is now available in multiple forms, including powder, capsules, and extracts.

In recent years, maca root has gained significant attention for its potential health benefits. It is often recognized as an adaptogen, a natural substance that helps the body adapt to stress and balance its functions. Maca root is rich in nutrients like vitamins, minerals, and antioxidants, which contribute to its therapeutic properties.

Some potential benefits associated with maca root include boosting energy levels, improving mood and mental well-being, enhancing sexual function and libido, supporting hormonal balance, and promoting overall vitality. It has also been studied for its potential effects on fertility, menopausal symptoms, and sports performance, among other areas.

As with any herbal remedy, it is essential to consult with a healthcare professional before incorporating maca root into your routine, especially if you have any underlying medical conditions or are taking medications. They can provide personalized guidance and ensure its safe and appropriate use.

In conclusion, maca root is a fascinating herb with a rich history and many potential health benefits. Its traditional use and increasing scientific interest make it an intriguing option for those seeking natural ways to support their well-being.

Case Studies on Maca Root

CASE STUDY #1

Menopause symptoms: A study published in the journal Menopause found that maca root may help alleviate symptoms of menopause, such as hot flashes and night sweats. The study involved 120 postmenopausal women who were randomly assigned to receive either maca root or a placebo for 12 weeks (about 3 months). At the end of the study, the women who received maca root reported a significant reduction in hot flashes and night sweats compared to those who received the placebo.

CASE STUDY #2

Sexual dysfunction: A study published in the journal CNS Neuroscience & Therapeutics found that maca root may help improve sexual dysfunction in women taking antidepressant medications. The study involved 45 women who were randomly assigned to receive either maca root or a placebo for eight weeks. At the end of the study, the women who received maca root reported a significant improvement in sexual function compared to those who received the placebo.

CASE STUDY #3

Energy and mood: A study published in the journal Evidence-Based Complementary and Alternative Medicine found that maca root may help improve energy and mood in postmenopausal women. The study involved 14 postmenopausal women who were given maca root for six weeks. At the end of the study, the women reported a significant improvement in energy levels and mood compared to their baseline levels.

CASE STUDY #4

Skin health: A study published in the journal International Journal of Cosmetic Science found that maca root may help improve skin health in women. The study involved 22 women who were given maca root for 12 weeks (about 3 months). At the end of the study, the women reported a significant improvement in skin elasticity, hydration, and texture compared to their baseline levels.

RECIPE 1

Maca Root "Strong Back" Smoothie

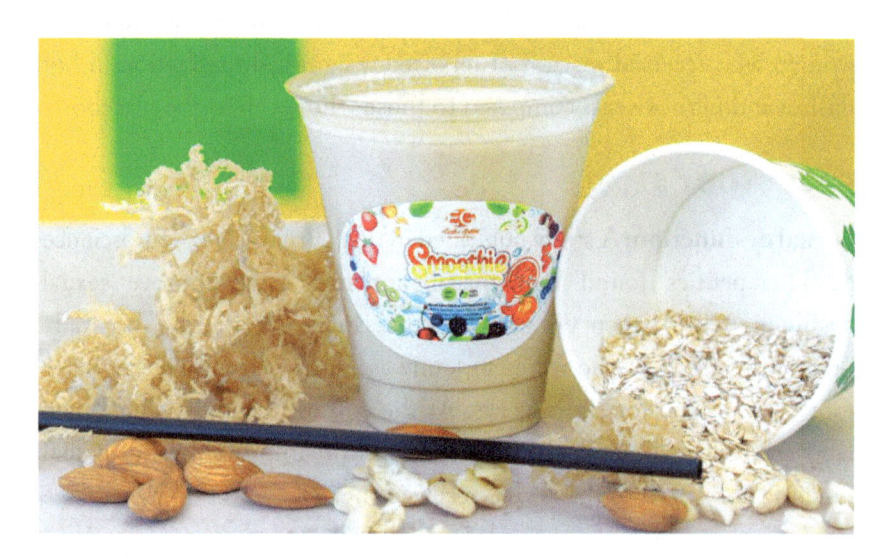

Ingredients:

- 1 frozen banana
- 1 cup almond milk
- 1/2 cup oats
- 1 tablespoon maca root powder
- 1/2 teaspoon vanilla extract
- 1/4 teaspoon ground cinnamon
- 1/4 teaspoon ground nutmeg
- 1 tablespoon sea moss gel
- ¼ cup of cashew
- 1 tablespoon agave (optional)

Instructions:

Add all ingredients to a blender.

Blend on high until smooth and creamy.

Taste and adjust sweetness with honey, if needed.

Pour into a glass and enjoy your delicious and nutritious Maca Root "Strong Back" Smoothie!

> Note: You can also add other healthy ingredients to this smoothie, such as spinach or kale for extra nutrition. Be sure to use high-quality maca root powder for the best flavor and health benefits.

RECIPE 2

Nutritious Maca Root Juice

Ingredients:

- 1 apple, chopped
- 1 pear, chopped
- 1/2 cucumber, chopped
- 1-inch piece of ginger, peeled and grated
- 1 tablespoon maca root powder
- 1 cup water

Instructions:

Add the chopped apple, pear, cucumber, and ginger to a juicer.

Juice the ingredients until smooth.

Pour the juice into a blender.

Add the maca root powder and water to the blender.

Blend on high until smooth and well-combined.

Pour the juice into a glass and enjoy your delicious and healthy Maca Root Juice!

> Note: You can adjust the ingredients to your liking and add more water if you prefer a thinner consistency. Be sure to use high-quality maca root powder for the best flavor and health benefits. You can also add other healthy ingredients such as lemon or lime juice for extra flavor and nutrition.

RECIPE 3

Maca Root Herbal Tea

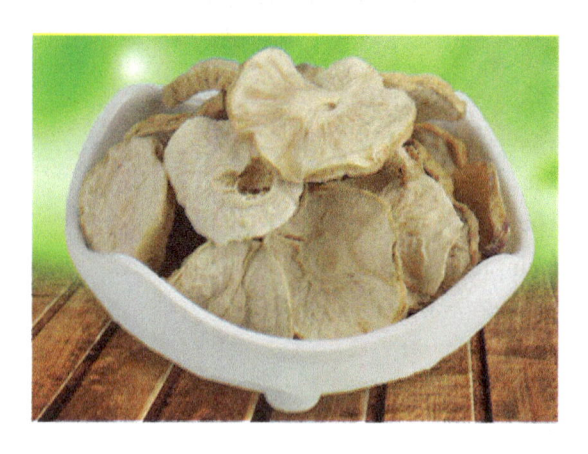

Ingredients:

- 1 teaspoon maca root powder
- 1 cup hot water
- 1 teaspoon agave (optional)

Instructions:

Add the maca root powder to a mug.

Pour hot water over the maca root powder.

Stir well until the maca root powder is dissolved. If desired, add honey to taste.

Let the tea cool for a few minutes before enjoying.

Note: You can adjust the amount of maca root powder to your liking and add honey depending on your preferred sweetness. Also, be sure to use high-quality maca root powder for the best flavor and health benefits.

HERB 8

Red Raspberry Leaf (Rubus idaeus) Herb

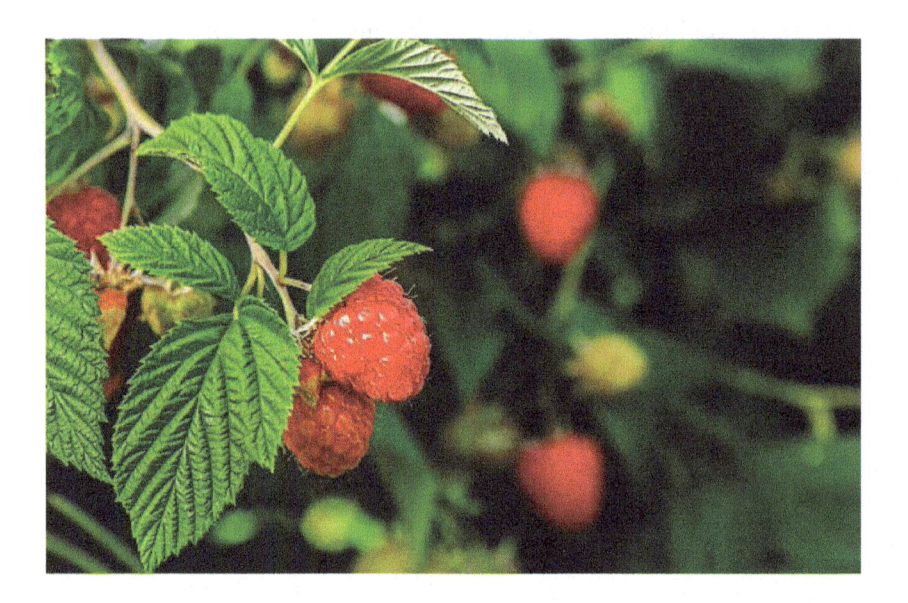

Red Raspberry Leaf, scientifically known as Rubus idaeus, is an herb that belongs to the Rosaceae family, which includes other familiar plants like roses and strawberries. The plant is native to Europe and certain parts of Asia but is now cultivated and widely grown in various regions worldwide.

The history of Red Raspberry Leaf stretches back centuries, and it has been used in traditional herbal medicine practices by diverse cultures. The ancient Greeks, Romans, and Native American tribes recognized and incorporated the plant's medicinal properties into their healing traditions.

During the Middle Ages, Red Raspberry Leaf gained popularity as a remedy for various ailments. It alleviated gastrointestinal issues, soothed sore throats, and supported women's reproductive health. The leaves were dried and brewed into teas or used as poultices for topical applications.

One of the primary uses of Red Raspberry Leaf throughout history has been its association with women's health, particularly during pregnancy and childbirth. It was highly regarded as a uterine tonic and was believed to strengthen the uterus, promote efficient contractions, and ease labor pains. Traditional midwives often recommended Red Raspberry Leaf tea to expectant mothers.

In addition to its role in supporting reproductive health, Red Raspberry Leaf has been valued for its potential benefits in other areas. It is often regarded as a rich source of vitamins, minerals, and antioxidants, including vitamin C, vitamin E, calcium, and magnesium. These nutrients contribute to its reputed nourishing and toning effects on the body.

Today, Red Raspberry Leaf remains a popular herb for women's health and is widely used during pregnancy and breastfeeding. It is also appreciated for its potential to support menstrual health and alleviate symptoms of premenstrual syndrome (P.M.S.). Red Raspberry Leaf is sometimes included in herbal formulations designed to promote overall well-being and support various bodily functions.

While Red Raspberry Leaf is considered safe for most individuals, it is advisable to consult a healthcare professional before using it, especially during pregnancy or if you have any underlying medical conditions. They can provide personalized advice based on your specific circumstances.

In conclusion, Red Raspberry Leaf is an herb with a long and storied history, particularly concerning women's health. Its traditional use and continued popularity today highlight its potential benefits in supporting reproductive health, menstrual wellness, and overall vitality.

Case Studies on Red Raspberry Leaf Case

STUDY #1

Menstrual cramps: A study published in the Journal of Midwifery & Women's Health found that red raspberry leaf may help reduce menstrual cramps. The study involved 55 women who were randomly assigned to receive either red raspberry leaf or a placebo for one menstrual cycle. At the end of the study, the women who received red raspberry leaf reported a significant reduction in menstrual cramps compared to those who received the placebo.

CASE STUDY #2

Labor and delivery: A study published in the Journal of Nurse-Midwifery found that red raspberry leaf may help shorten labor and reduce the need for interventions during childbirth. The study involved 192 women who were randomly assigned to receive either red raspberry leaf or a placebo during pregnancy. At the end of the study, the women who received red raspberry leaf had a shorter second stage of labor and were less likely to need interventions such as forceps delivery or cesarean section.

CASE STUDY #3

Breastfeeding: A study published in the Journal of Human Lactation found that red raspberry leaf may help increase breast milk production in postpartum women. The study involved 120 postpartum women who were randomly assigned to receive either red raspberry leaf or a placebo for two weeks. At the end of the study, the women who received red raspberry leaf had a significant increase in breast milk production compared to those who received the placebo.

CASE STUDY #4

Digestive health: A study published in the journal Planta Medica found that red raspberry leaf may help alleviate diarrhea and other digestive symptoms. The study involved 60 people with diarrhea who were randomly assigned to receive either red raspberry leaf or a placebo. At the end of the study, the group that received red raspberry leaf reported a significant reduction in diarrhea and other digestive symptoms compared to the placebo group.

RECIPE 1

Red Raspberry Leaf Herbal Tea

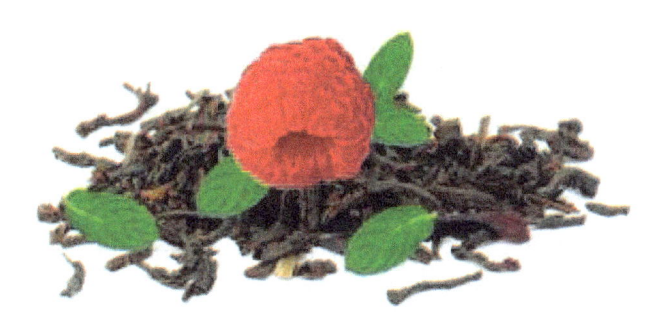

Ingredients:

- 1 tablespoon dried red raspberry leaves or 2-3 fresh raspberry leaves
- 1 cup boiling water
- agave or lemon (optional)

Instructions:

Place the dried or fresh raspberry leaves in a tea strainer or infuser.

Pour the boiling water over the leaves.

Let it steep for 5-10 minutes, depending on how strong your tea is.

Remove the tea strainer or infuser and discard the leaves.

If desired, add honey or lemon for flavor.

Enjoy your delicious and healthy Red Raspberry Leaf Herbal Tea!

RECIPE 2

Red Raspberry Smoothie

Ingredients:

- 1 cup frozen raspberries
- 1/2 cup unsweetened vanilla almond milk (or any other type of milk)
- 1/2 cup vanilla Greek yogurt
- 1/2 banana
- 1 tablespoon honey
- 1 teaspoon vanilla extract
- 1/2 cup ice

Instructions:

Add all ingredients to a blender.

Blend until smooth and creamy.

If the smoothie is too thick, add more almond milk or water.

Pour the smoothie into a glass and enjoy immediately.

Note: You can adjust the amount of honey to your liking and add ice depending on how thick your smoothie is. You can also use fresh raspberries instead of frozen ones, but frozen raspberries give the smoothie a nice texture and make it cold and refreshing.

RECIPE 3

Refreshing and healthy Red Raspberry Juice

Ingredients:

- 2 cups fresh or frozen raspberries
- 1/2 cup water
- 1/4 cup honey or agave syrup
- 1 lemon, juiced

Instructions:

Add the raspberries and water to a blender and blend until smooth.

Pour the mixture through a fine mesh strainer to remove any seeds or pulp.

Add the honey or agave syrup and lemon juice to the strained raspberry juice and stir until well combined.

Taste and adjust sweetness with more honey or agave syrup if desired.

Chill the juice in the refrigerator for at least 30 minutes.

Serve in glasses with ice cubes and garnish with fresh raspberries or lemon slices.

HERB 9

Wild Yam (Dioscorea Villosa) Herb

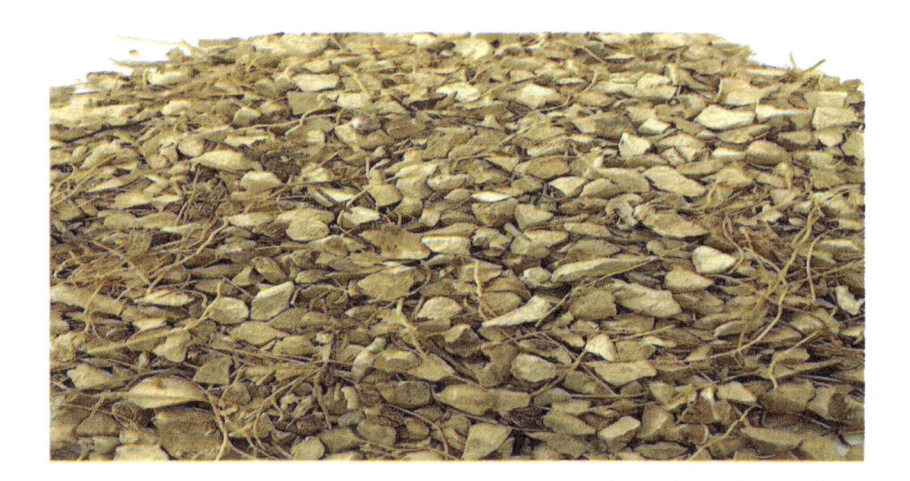

Wild Yam, scientifically known as Dioscorea villosa, is a perennial vine that belongs to the Dioscoreaceae family. It is native to North America, particularly the eastern and central regions of the continent. The plant has a long history of traditional use by various indigenous cultures for its medicinal properties.

The indigenous tribes of North America, such as the Cherokee and Iroquois, were among the first to recognize and utilize the therapeutic potential of Wild Yam. They harvested the plant's tubers, which are the underground parts of the vine, and used them for various medicinal purposes. Wild Yam was valued for its potential to alleviate gastrointestinal issues, menstrual discomfort, and general pain.

In the late 19th and early 20th centuries, Wild Yam gained popularity in traditional herbal medicine practices, particularly for its association with women's health. It was commonly used to support reproductive health and address menstrual complaints. The herb was believed to have estrogenic properties and was used as a natural alternative to hormonal therapies.

The name "Wild Yam" can be attributed to the plant's resemblance to true yams, starchy tuberous roots commonly used as a food source. However, it is essential to note that Wild Yam is unrelated to the edible yam varieties and does not have the same nutritional profile.

The active compounds found in Wild Yam, including diosgenin, are believed to contribute to its medicinal properties. Diosgenin is a precursor to various hormones, including progesterone, and has been the subject of scientific research exploring its potential therapeutic applications.

Today, Wild Yam is often included in herbal formulations designed to support women's health, particularly during menopause and menstruation. It is reputed to help balance hormone levels, alleviate menstrual discomfort, and support overall reproductive wellness. Additionally, Wild Yam is sometimes used topically in creams or ointments for skin conditions.

While Wild Yam is considered safe for most individuals when used appropriately, it is advisable to consult a healthcare professional before using it, especially if you have any underlying medical conditions or are taking medications. They can provide guidance and ensure its safe and effective use.

In summary, Wild Yam has a rich history rooted in traditional indigenous medicine and has been valued for its potential benefits in supporting women's health. Its historical use and continued utilization in modern herbal medicine highlight its potential as a natural remedy for menstrual discomfort and reproductive wellness.

Case Studies on Wild Yam

CASE STUDY #1

Menopausal Symptoms: A study published in the Journal of Nurse Midwifery examined the effects of a wild yam cream on menopausal symptoms in a group of women. The researchers found that the cream was effective in reducing the frequency and severity of hot flashes, night sweats, and vaginal dryness.

CASE STUDY #2

Dysmenorrhea: A small study published in the Journal of Complementary and Integrative Medicine examined the effects of a wild yam cream on dysmenorrhea (painful menstruation). The researchers found that the cream was effective in reducing pain and other symptoms associated with dysmenorrhea.

CASE STUDY #3

Colitis: A study published in the Journal of Ethnopharmacology examined the effects of a wild yam extract on colitis in rats. The researchers found that the extract was effective in reducing inflammation and improving the overall health of the animals' colons.

CASE STUDY #4

Cholesterol Levels: A study published in the Journal of Medicinal Food examined the effects of a wild yam extract on cholesterol levels in a group of overweight adults. The researchers found that the extract was effective in reducing total cholesterol and LDL cholesterol levels.

RECIPE 1

Wild Yam Herbal Tea

Ingredients:

- 1-2 teaspoons of dried wild yam root
- 1 cup of water

Instructions:

Bring the water to a boil in a small pot or kettle.

Add the dried wild yam root to a tea infuser or a small muslin bag.

Place the infuser or bag in a cup.

Pour the boiling water over the infuser or bag.

Cover the cup and let the tea steep for 5-10 minutes.

RECIPE 2

Wild Yam Smoothie

Ingredients:

- 1 banana
- 1/2 cup frozen berries (e.g., blueberries, strawberries, raspberries)
- 1/2 cup almond milk
- 1 tablespoon wild yam powder
- 1/2 teaspoon cinnamon
- 1/2 teaspoon vanilla extract
- 1 tablespoon honey (optional)

Instructions:

Add all ingredients to a blender.

Blend until smooth and creamy.

If the mixture is too thick, add more almond milk.

Taste the smoothie and add honey if needed for sweetness.

Pour the smoothie into a glass and enjoy!

> Note: Pregnant women should avoid using wild yam as it may stimulate the uterus. If you are taking medication or have a medical condition, it is best to consult with a healthcare provider before using wild yam or any herbal supplements.

RECIPE 3

Wild Yam Juice

Ingredients:

- 1 medium-sized sweet potato
- 1 medium-sized carrot
- 1 inch piece of fresh ginger
- 1 tablespoon wild yam powder
- 1/2 cup water
- 1/2 cup ice

Instructions:

Wash and peel the sweet potato, carrot, and ginger.

Cut them into small pieces that can fit into a juicer.

Put the sweet potato, carrot, and ginger through a juicer to extract the juice.

In a blender, mix the wild yam powder with water to create a smooth paste. Add the ice to the blender and blend until the ice is crushed.

Pour the sweet potato, carrot, and ginger juice into the blender with the wild yam paste and blend again until well combined.

Taste the juice and adjust the sweetness by adding honey or other sweeteners if needed.

Pour the juice into a glass and serve immediately.

> Note: Pregnant women should avoid using wild yam as it may stimulate the uterus. If you are taking medication or have a medical condition, it is best to consult with a healthcare provider before using wild yam or any herbal supplement.

BONUS HERB #1
Burdock root (Arctium lappa)

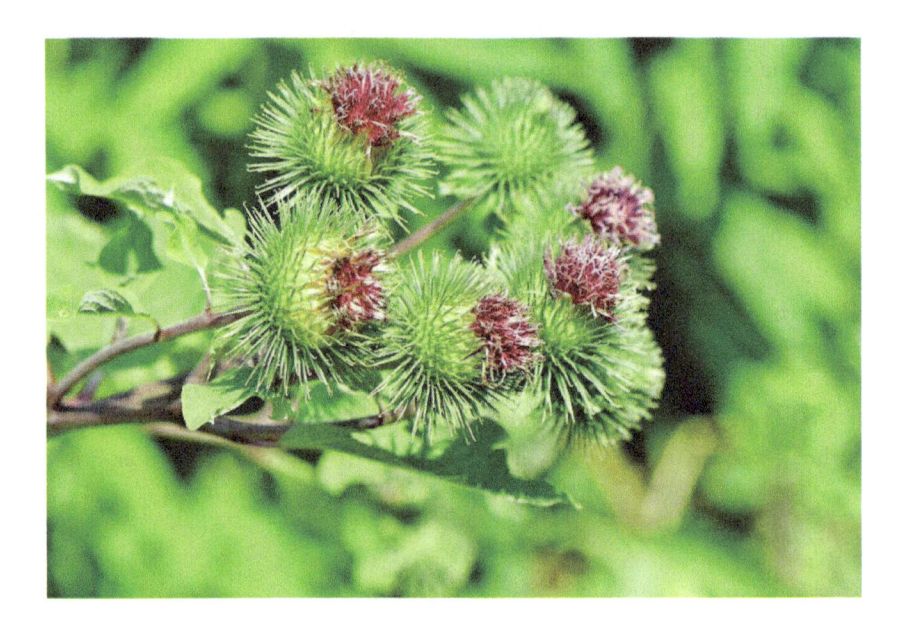

Burdock, scientifically known as Arctium lappa, is a biennial herbaceous plant that belongs to the Asteraceae family. It is native to Europe and Asia but is now widely distributed and naturalized in various parts of the world. Burdock is known for its distinctive appearance, with large, heart-shaped leaves and prickly burrs that stick to clothing or animal fur, aiding in seed dispersal.

The history of Burdock stretches back centuries, and it has been valued for its culinary and medicinal properties. In traditional herbal medicine, Burdock has been used as a diuretic, blood purifier, and digestive aid. Its roots, leaves, and seeds have been employed for various therapeutic purposes.

Historically, Burdock was widely used in traditional Chinese medicine, known as Niu Bang Zi. Its seeds were particularly prized for their potential to support respiratory health and clear heat from the body. In Japanese traditional medicine, Burdock was called Gobo, and the roots were used as a blood purifier to support healthy skin.

In Western herbal medicine, Burdock has been regarded as a "blood cleanser" used to support liver health and promote healthy digestion. It was believed to help eliminate toxins from the body and support overall wellness.

Burdock has also been used as a culinary ingredient, especially in Asian cuisines. The root is often used in stir-fries, soups, and teas, while the young leaves are occasionally used as vegetables. Burdock root has a slightly sweet and earthy flavor, making it a unique addition to various dishes.

Burdock's roots contain many active compounds, including inulin, polyphenols, and volatile oils. These components contribute to its potential health benefits. Inulin, for instance, is a prebiotic fiber that can support the growth of beneficial gut bacteria and promote digestive health.

Today, Burdock is still utilized in herbal medicine and is often included in herbal formulations and teas to support detoxification, promote healthy skin, and maintain overall well-being. It is also an ingredient in natural skincare products because it can soothe skin conditions like eczema and acne.

As with any herbal remedy, it is essential to consult with a healthcare professional before using Burdock, especially if you have any underlying health conditions or are taking medications. They can guide appropriate dosage and ensure its safe use.

In summary, Burdock has a rich history in traditional medicine, spanning diverse cultures and regions. Its versatile uses, both culinary and medicinal, highlight its historical significance.

Whether consumed as a food or herbal remedy, Burdock offers potential health benefits. It continues to be valued for supporting liver function, promoting healthy digestion, and contributing to overall well-being.

Case Studies on Burdock Root

CASE STUDY #1

A study published in the journal Phytotherapy Research found that burdock root extract may help lower blood sugar levels in people with type 2 diabetes. The study involved 42 participants given either burdock root extract or a placebo for 28 days (about 4 weeks). The researchers found that those who took the burdock root extract had significantly lower fasting blood sugar levels compared to the placebo group.

CASE STUDY #2

Another study published in the Journal of Ethnopharmacology found that burdock root extract may have anti-inflammatory effects. The study involved testing the extract on human white blood cells in vitro, and the researchers found it could suppress the production of inflammatory compounds.

CASE STUDY #3

A study published in the Journal of Medicinal Food found that burdock root may have anticancer properties. The study involved testing burdock root extract on human colon cancer cells in vitro, and the researchers found that it could inhibit the growth and spread of the cancer cells.

CASE STUDY #4

A study published in the Journal of Cosmetic Dermatology found that burdock root extract may help improve the appearance of acne-prone skin. The study involved 20 participants who applied a burdock root extract cream to their faces twice daily for 8 weeks (about 2 months).

The researchers found that the participants had significant improvements in their acne symptoms, including a reduction in the number of acne lesions and improved skin texture.

BONUS RECIPE 1

Burdock Root Herbal Tea (Blood Cleanser)

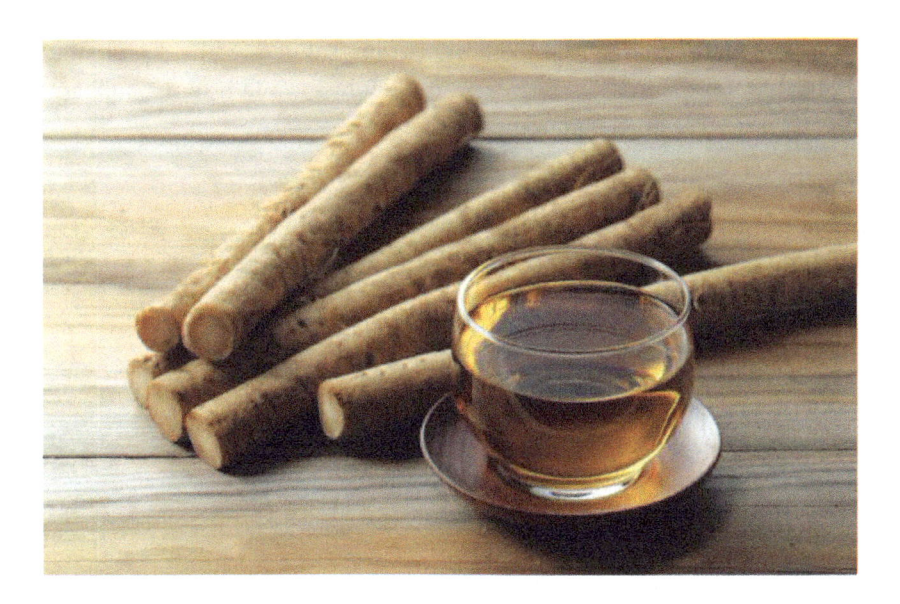

Ingredients:

- 1-2 teaspoons dried burdock root
- 2 cups water
- Optional: honey, lemon, or other natural sweeteners

Instructions:

Bring 2 cups of water to a boil in a small saucepan.

Add 1-2 teaspoons of dried burdock root to the boiling water.

Reduce the heat to low and let the burdock root simmer for about 10-15 minutes.

Strain the tea through a fine mesh strainer to remove the burdock root.

If desired, add honey, lemon, or other natural sweeteners to taste.

Serve hot and enjoy your homemade burdock root tea!

Note: You can also use fresh burdock root instead of dried burdock root. Simply wash the root thoroughly, slice it thinly, and add it to the boiling water instead of dried burdock root.

BONUS RECIPE 2

Herbal Tea Potent Support Formula to Balance the Hormone

Ingredients:

- 1 tablespoon red clover flowers
- 1 tablespoon vitex berries
- 1 tablespoon raspberry leaf
- 1 tablespoon dong quai root
- 1 tablespoon black cohosh root
- 1 tablespoon burdock root
- 4 cups water

Instructions:

In a medium-sized pot, add the water and bring it to a boil.

Reduce heat to low and add all the dried herbs to the pot.

Cover the pot and let the herbs steep for about 15-20 minutes.

After 15-20 minutes, turn off the heat and strain the tea into a cup.

You can sweeten the tea with honey or another natural sweetener if you would like.

Enjoy your hormone balancing tea!

Note: This tea recipe is meant to be consumed in moderation and is not intended to diagnose, treat, or cure any medical condition. If you have a medical condition or are taking medication, it is best to consult with a healthcare provider before using any herbal supplements. Also, some of these herbs may not be suitable for pregnant or breastfeeding women, so it is important to check with a healthcare provider before using this tea.

BONUS RECIPE 3

Delicious Burdock Root Smoothie

Ingredients:

- 1 cup cold pressed red apple juice
- 1/2 cup frozen kale
- ½ cup frozen spinach
- ½ cup frozen pineapples
- ½ cup frozen strawberries

- 1/2-inch fresh ginger, peeled and grated
- 1 teaspoon dried burdock root powder

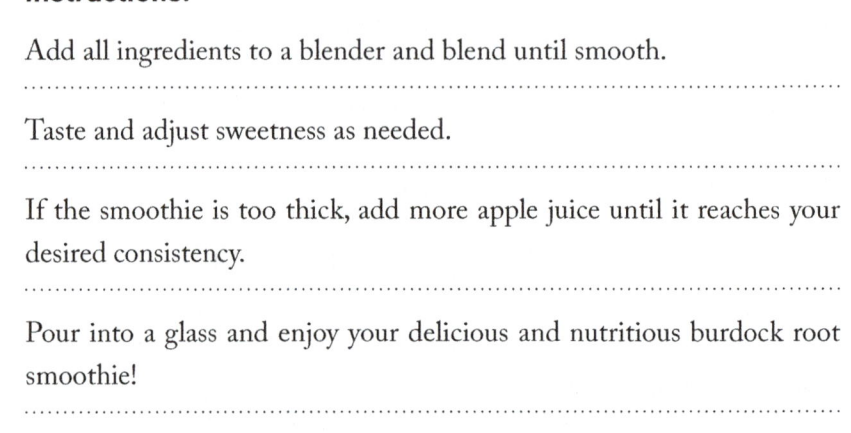

Instructions:

Add all ingredients to a blender and blend until smooth.

Taste and adjust sweetness as needed.

If the smoothie is too thick, add more apple juice until it reaches your desired consistency.

Pour into a glass and enjoy your delicious and nutritious burdock root smoothie!

Note: If you do not have burdock root powder, you can use fresh burdock root. Wash and peel the root, then chop it into small pieces and blend it with the other ingredients.

BONUS RECIPE 4

Delicious Burdock Root Juice

Ingredients:

- 2-3 fresh burdock roots, washed and peeled
- 1-2 carrots, washed and peeled
- ½ beet, washed and cored
- 1 lemon, peeled
- 1-inch piece of ginger, peeled
- Water

Instructions:

Wash and peel the burdock roots and carrots and chop them into small pieces.

Cut the beet into small chunks.

Peel the lemon and ginger.

Add all ingredients to a juicer and process until smooth.

If the juice is too thick, add some water to thin it out.

Pour the juice into a glass and enjoy your homemade burdock root juice!

> Note: If you do not have a juicer, you can use a blender and strain the juice through a fine mesh strainer or cheesecloth to remove any solids. You can also adjust the ingredients to suit your taste preferences, adding ginger or lemon juice as desired.

BONUS HERB #2
Sea Moss (Chondrus crispus) AKA Irish Moss

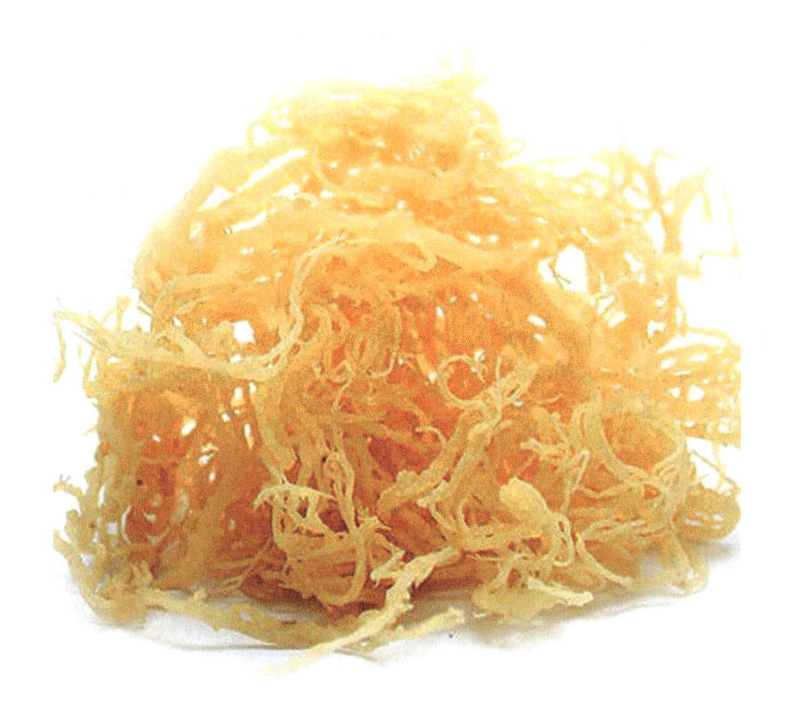

In the depths of the calm, clear waters of the Atlantic Ocean, there existed a humble plant with a remarkable history. This plant, called Sea Moss or Irish Moss, held within its delicate fronds a wealth of nourishment and healing properties that would captivate the world.

Sea Moss, scientifically known as Chondrus crispus, has a history as ancient as the ocean. It has been cherished for centuries, originating from the rocky shores of the North Atlantic, particularly along the coasts of

Ireland, Scotland, and other regions with similar maritime climates. The people who inhabited these lands discovered the incredible benefits of this marine treasure and incorporated it into their diets and traditional medicine practices.

Throughout history, Sea Moss has been revered for its outstanding nutritional profile. It is rich in essential minerals such as iodine, potassium, calcium, magnesium, and iron, vital for maintaining optimal health and supporting bodily functions. This natural wonder also contains various vitamins, including vitamins A, C, E, and B, contributing to overall well-being. Sea Moss provides 92 of the 102 minerals and nutrients our body requires. Combine sea moss, burdock root, and bladderwrack herbs, and you will get the 102 minerals and nutrients your body needs not to get sleepy or tired.

One of the most notable benefits of Sea Moss lies in its ability to support respiratory health. The plant contains a gummy substance that, when consumed, forms a soft gel-like consistency that coats the throat and soothes irritated mucous membranes. This property has made Sea Moss a popular remedy for alleviating respiratory conditions such as coughs, sore throats, and even respiratory infections.

But Sea Moss's benefits continue beyond there. It is also known for its potential to support digestion and gut health. The high fiber content of Sea Moss helps promote healthy digestion, aiding in regulating bowel movements and preventing constipation, and suppressing the appetite. Furthermore, the plant's natural prebiotic properties can support the growth of beneficial gut bacteria, contributing to a healthy gut microbiome.

In addition to its nutritional and digestive benefits, Sea Moss has been praised for its potential to boost immune function and provide anti-inflammatory properties. Its great mineral content and antioxidant compounds may help strengthen the immune system and protect against oxidative stress, thus promoting overall wellness and vitality.

Throughout the ages, Sea Moss has played a vital role in traditional medicine and culinary practices, with various cultures incorporating it into their diets in diverse ways. From using it as a thickening agent in soups and stews to blending it into smoothies and incorporating it into desserts, the versatility of Sea Moss has made it a beloved ingredient in countless recipes worldwide.

Today, the story of Sea Moss continues to unfold. Its popularity has surged as more people rediscover the hidden gems of nature's bounty. Whether enjoyed for its nutritional value, healing properties, or culinary delights, Sea Moss remains a testament to the wonders of the ocean and the timeless wisdom of ancient traditions.

So, dive into the world of Sea Moss, embrace its rich history, and let its benefits wash over you, revitalizing your body, mind, and spirit. As you incorporate this remarkable plant into your life, may you experience the transformative power of nature's gifts, and may your journey be one of vibrant health and well-being.

Case Studies on SEA MOSS

CASE STUDY # 1:

Patient: Sarah, a 35-year-old female

Symptoms: Sarah had recurrent respiratory infections, including a persistent cough, sore throat, and congestion. These symptoms significantly affected her quality of life and made it challenging to perform daily activities.

Treatment: Sarah started incorporating Sea Moss into her diet regularly. She consumed Sea Moss gel by blending it into her morning smoothies and adding it to soups and stews.

Results: After two months of consistent Sea Moss consumption, Sarah noticed a significant improvement in her respiratory health. Her cough became less frequent and severe, and her sore throat symptoms diminished. She experienced fewer instances of congestion and felt more energized overall.

CASE STUDY # 2:

Patient: Michael, a 45-year-old male

Symptoms: Michael had been dealing with occasional constipation and irregular bowel movements. He also experienced bloating and discomfort after meals, which affected his overall digestion.

Treatment: Michael incorporated Sea Moss into his diet as a Sea Moss-infused smoothie every morning. He also consumed Sea Moss gel as a natural thickening agent in his soups and sauces.

Results: After four weeks of including Sea Moss in his daily routine, Michael noticed significant improvements in his digestive health. His bowel movements became regular, and he experienced less bloating and discomfort after meals. He reported feeling lighter and more comfortable in his digestive system.

CASE STUDY # 3:

Patient: Emily, a 28-year-old female

Symptoms: Emily had been dealing with frequent colds and flu-like symptoms, often catching every bug. Her weak immune system made it difficult for her to stay healthy, impacting her work and personal life.

Treatment: Emily started consuming Sea Moss gel daily, either on her own or mixed with other nutritious ingredients like citrus fruits and ginger. She also incorporated Sea Moss into her baking, using it as a binder in healthy snack bars.

Results: After three months of consistent Sea Moss consumption, Emily experienced a noticeable boost in her immune function. She reported fewer incidences of getting sick and recovering faster when she did catch a cold. She felt more resilient and better equipped to fight off infections.

Sea Moss Gel Recipe

Ingredients:

- 1 cup dried sea moss (Irish moss) (Make sure you are using potent sea moss)
- 2 cups filtered water

Instructions:

Rinse the dried sea moss thoroughly under running water to remove any debris or salt.

Soak the sea moss in a bowl of filtered water for 24 hours. This will help it rehydrate and soften.

After soaking, the sea moss will have expanded in size. Drain the water from the bowl. Transfer the soaked sea moss to a blender.

Add 2 cups of filtered water to the blender. You can adjust the amount of water depending on how thick or thin you want your gel to be.

Blend on high speed until the mixture becomes smooth and gel-like in consistency. This usually takes a few minutes.

Pour the sea moss gel into a clean glass jar with an airtight lid.

Store the jar in the refrigerator for at least 4 hours or overnight to allow the gel to set and thicken.

Once chilled, the sea moss gel is ready to be used.

> Note: Sea moss gel can be stored in the refrigerator for up to 2 weeks. It may naturally thicken over time, but you can simply stir it or add a little water to adjust the consistency as needed.

Enjoy your homemade sea moss gel! It can be used as a nutritious addition to smoothies, juices, desserts, or as a thickening agent in various recipes. Remember to incorporate it into your daily routine for its potential health benefits and hormone-balancing properties.

Sea Moss Bonus Smoothie Recipe # 1

Ingredients:

- 1 ripe mango, peeled and pitted
- 1 cup pineapple chunks
- 1 small cucumber, peeled and chopped
- 1 tablespoon sea moss gel
- 1 cup coconut water
- 1 tablespoon lime juice
- Handful of fresh mint leaves
- Ice cubes (optional)

Instructions:

Chop the ripe mango, pineapple chunks, and cucumber into smaller pieces.

In a blender, add the chopped mango, pineapple chunks, cucumber, sea moss gel, coconut water, lime juice, and fresh mint leaves.

If desired, add a few ice cubes for a chilled smoothie.

Blend on high speed until all the ingredients are well combined and the smoothie reaches a smooth and creamy consistency.

Taste the smoothie and adjust the sweetness or tanginess by adding more lime juice or a natural sweetener like honey or agave syrup if desired.

Pour the sea moss smoothie into a glass or jar.

Garnish with a sprig of fresh mint leaves for an extra touch of freshness.

Sip and enjoy your refreshing sea moss smoothie!

This tropical-inspired smoothie combines the goodness of mango, pineapple, cucumber, and sea moss to create a delightful and refreshing blend. It is a perfect way to incorporate sea moss into your diet while enjoying the flavors of the tropics. Cheers to your health and well- being!

Sea Moss Bonus Smoothie Recipe # 2

Ingredients:

- 1 ripe banana
- 1 cup frozen mixed berries (strawberries, blueberries, raspberries)
- 1 cup almond milk (or any plant-based milk of your choice)
- 1 tablespoon sea moss gel
- 1 tablespoon honey or maple syrup (optional for added sweetness)
- 1 teaspoon vanilla extract (optional for flavor)

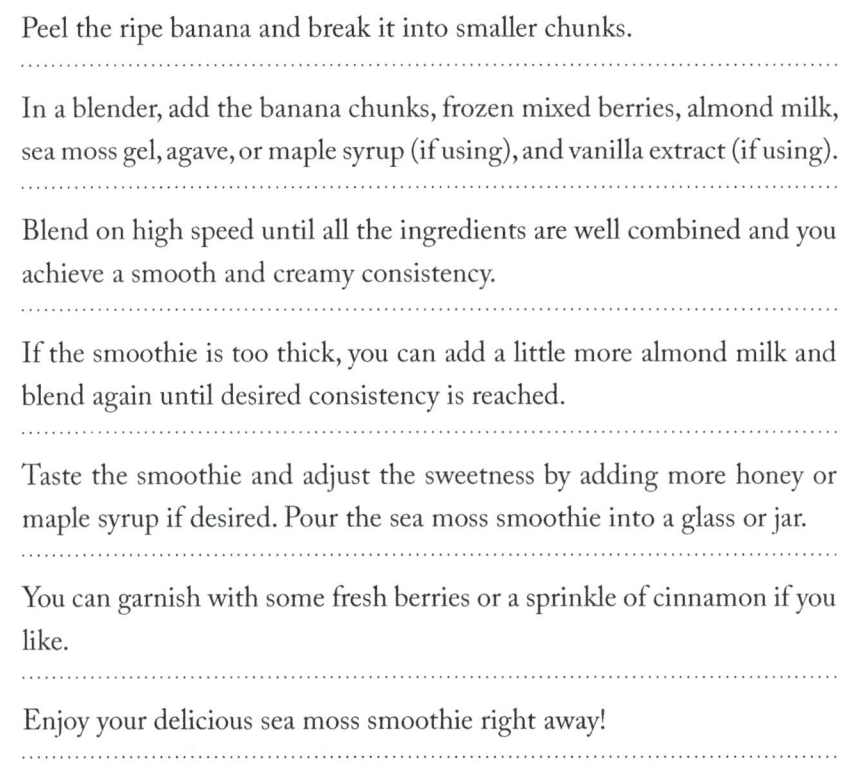

Instructions:

Peel the ripe banana and break it into smaller chunks.

In a blender, add the banana chunks, frozen mixed berries, almond milk, sea moss gel, agave, or maple syrup (if using), and vanilla extract (if using).

Blend on high speed until all the ingredients are well combined and you achieve a smooth and creamy consistency.

If the smoothie is too thick, you can add a little more almond milk and blend again until desired consistency is reached.

Taste the smoothie and adjust the sweetness by adding more honey or maple syrup if desired. Pour the sea moss smoothie into a glass or jar.

You can garnish with some fresh berries or a sprinkle of cinnamon if you like.

Enjoy your delicious sea moss smoothie right away!

This smoothie is not only tasty but also packed with nutrients from the sea moss and mixed berries. It can be a powerful addition to your daily routine for supporting hormonal balance and overall well-being. Cheers to a healthy and delicious treat!

EATING THE RIGHT FOODS, FRUITS, AND VEGETABLES FOR HORMONE IMBALANCES

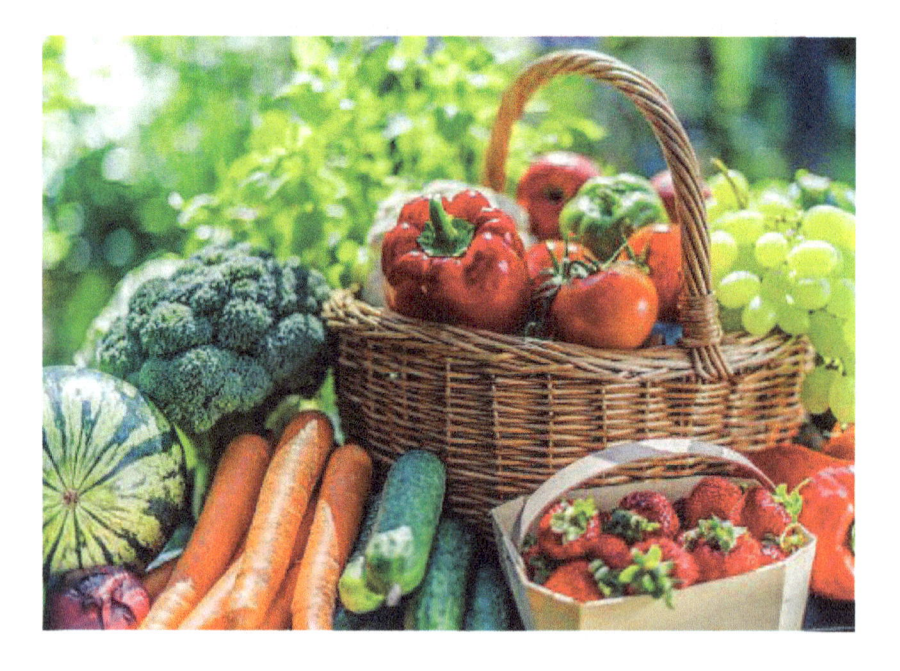

In this part of the book, you will learn about juicing and the best foods, fruits, and vegetables to consume when suffering from hormone imbalances.

Maintaining a healthy and balanced diet is crucial for women with hormone imbalances. Eating various nutrient-dense foods, including fruits, vegetables, whole grains, lean protein, and healthy fats, can help regulate hormone levels, reduce inflammation, and support overall health. Let us list some of the best foods, fruits, and vegetables that women with hormone imbalances should eat:

Leafy greens: Kale, spinach, collard greens, and other leafy greens are rich in vitamins, minerals, and antioxidants that support hormone balance.

Cruciferous vegetables: Broccoli, cauliflower, cabbage, and Brussels sprouts contain compounds that help to regulate estrogen levels and reduce the risk of breast cancer.

Berries: Blueberries, raspberries, strawberries, and other berries are high in antioxidants and fiber, which can help to regulate blood sugar and reduce inflammation.

Citrus fruits: Oranges, grapefruits, lemons, and limes are rich in vitamin C, which supports hormone production and immune function.

Avocado: Avocado is an excellent source of healthy fats, which can help to regulate hormone levels and reduce inflammation.

Nuts and seeds: Almonds, walnuts, chia seeds, and flaxseeds are all high in healthy fats, fiber, and protein, which can help to regulate hormone levels and support overall health.

Whole grains: Whole grains like quinoa, brown rice, and oats are rich in fiber and nutrients that help regulate blood sugar and support hormone balance.

Legumes: Beans, lentils, and chickpeas are all excellent sources of protein and fiber, which can help to regulate blood sugar and support hormone balance.

Fermented foods: Fermented foods like yogurt, kefir, and sauerkraut contain probiotics, which can help to support gut health and hormone balance.

Incorporating these foods into your diet and eating a well-balanced, nutrient-dense diet, women with hormone imbalances, can support their overall health and reduce the risk of hormonal ailments.

The Benefits of Juicing Fruits & Vegetables for Hormone Imbalances

Juicing fruits and vegetables can be a powerful tool in addressing hormone imbalances and restoring balance in your body. Here's how juicing can help you on your journey to hormonal health over 30 days (about 4 and a half weeks):

Nutrient Density: Fresh fruits and vegetables contain essential vitamins, minerals, and antioxidants that support hormonal balance. Juicing allows you to consume a concentrated dose of these nutrients, providing your body with the building blocks for hormone production and regulation.

Detoxification: Many hormone imbalances are caused or exacerbated by the accumulation of toxins in the body. Juicing acts as a natural detoxifier, helping to eliminate toxins and promote the proper functioning of your endocrine system. The abundance of antioxidants in fruits and vegetables helps neutralize harmful free radicals and support liver detoxification.

Phytonutrients: Fruits and vegetables contain potent plant compounds called phytonutrients. These compounds have been shown to have hormone-balancing effects and can help reduce inflammation, improve cellular communication, and support overall hormonal health. Juicing allows for easy absorption of these phytonutrients, maximizing their benefits.

Blood Sugar Regulation: Balanced blood sugar levels are crucial for hormonal health. Juicing vegetables and low-glycemic fruits can help stabilize blood sugar levels and prevent spikes and crashes that can disrupt hormone balance. This is especially important for insulin resistance and polycystic ovary syndrome (PCOS).

Gut Health: A healthy gut plays a vital role in hormonal balance. Fruits and vegetables are fiber- rich, nourishing beneficial gut bacteria and supporting a healthy digestive system. Juicing can provide a concentrated source of gut-friendly fiber, aiding digestion and nutrient absorption and eliminating waste and excess hormones.

Hormone-Supportive Ingredients: Certain fruits and vegetables have specific properties that support hormonal balance. For example, cruciferous vegetables like broccoli and kale contain compounds that assist in estrogen metabolism. Citrus fruits are rich in vitamin C, which aids in progesterone production. Incorporating these hormone-supportive ingredients into your juices can target specific imbalances and promote overall hormonal health.

Balanced Nutrition: Juicing allows you to easily consume various fruits and vegetables, ensuring a balanced intake of essential nutrients. A diverse and nutrient-rich diet is vital in supporting hormonal balance, as different vitamins and minerals play specific roles in hormone synthesis and regulation.

APRIL HEATH-WHITE, M.S., B.S., A.A.

It is important to note that juicing should not replace a well-rounded diet but rather complement it. Incorporating fresh juices into your daily routine, along with whole foods, can boost your hormonal health.

RECIPE 1

Quinoa and Kale Salad

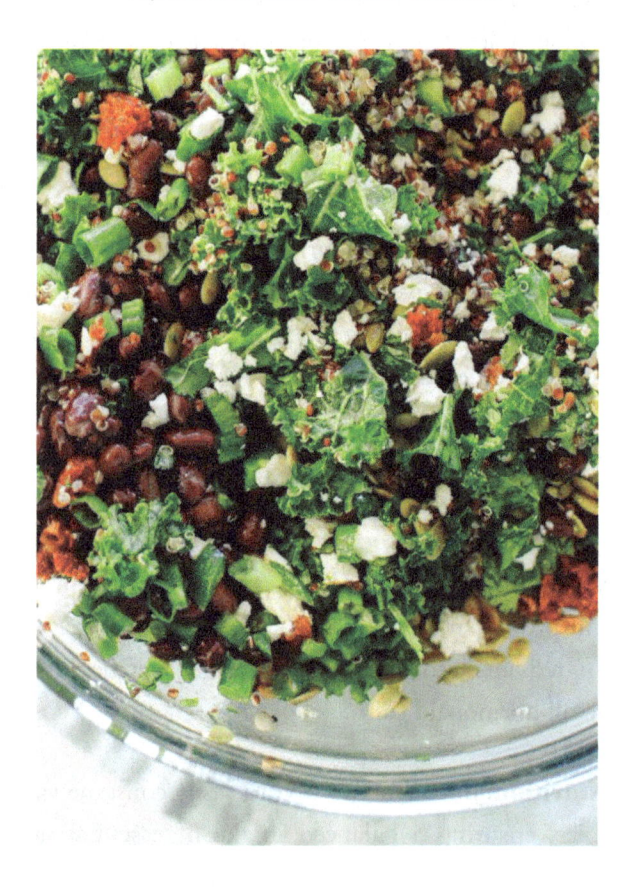

Ingredients:

- 1 cup quinoa, rinsed
- 2 cups vegetable broth

- 1 tablespoon olive oil
- 1 bunch kale, stems removed and chopped
- 1/2 cup chopped walnuts
- 1/2 cup dried cranberries
- 1/4 cup crumbled Daiya vegan cheese
- Salt and pepper to taste

Instructions:

In a medium saucepan, combine the quinoa and vegetable broth and bring to a boil.

Reduce the heat to low, cover the pot, and simmer for 15-20 minutes, or until the quinoa is tender.

In a large skillet, heat the olive oil over medium heat.

Add the kale and sauté for 3-4 minutes, or until wilted.

In a large bowl, combine the cooked quinoa, sautéed kale, chopped walnuts, dried cranberries, and crumbled Daiya vegan cheese.

Toss to combine and season with salt and pepper to taste.

Serve warm or chilled.

APRIL HEATH-WHITE, M.S., B.S., A.A.

RECIPE 3

Lentil Soup

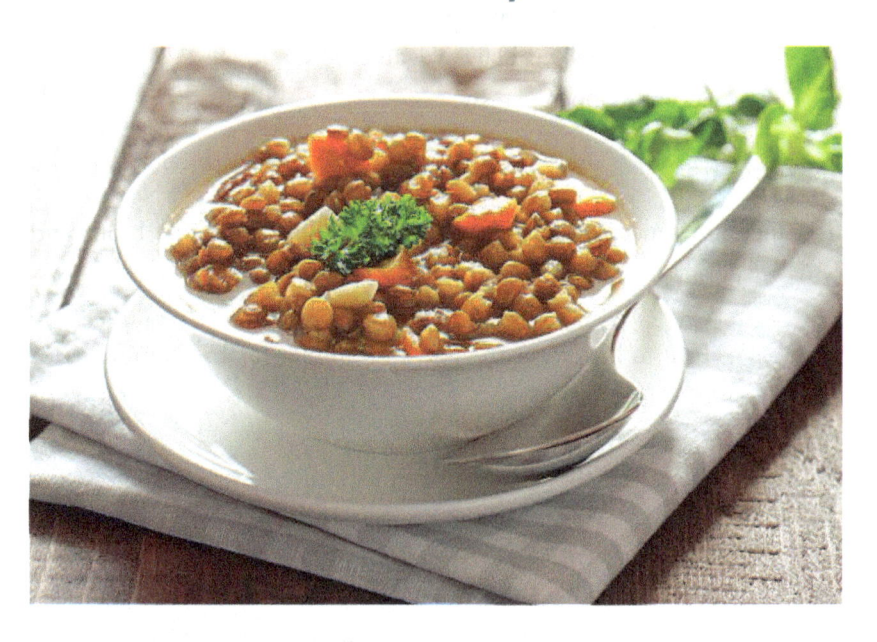

Ingredients:

- 1 cup red lentils
- 1 tablespoon olive oil
- 1 onion, chopped
- 2 cloves garlic, minced
- 2 teaspoons ground cumin
- 1 teaspoon ground coriander
- 4 cups vegetable broth
- 1 can diced tomatoes
- 1 cup chopped carrots
- 1 cup chopped celery
- Salt and pepper to taste

Instructions:

Rinse the lentils in a fine mesh strainer and set aside.

Heat the olive oil in a large pot over medium heat.

Add the onion and sauté for 3-4 minutes, or until softened.

Add the garlic, cumin, and coriander and sauté for another minute.

Add the vegetable broth, diced tomatoes, lentils, carrots, and celery.

Bring the soup to a boil, then reduce the heat to low and simmer for 20-25 minutes, or until the lentils are tender.

Season with salt and pepper to taste.

Serve hot.

APRIL HEATH-WHITE, M.S., B.S., A.A.

RECIPE 4

Roasted Sweet Potato and Brussels Sprouts

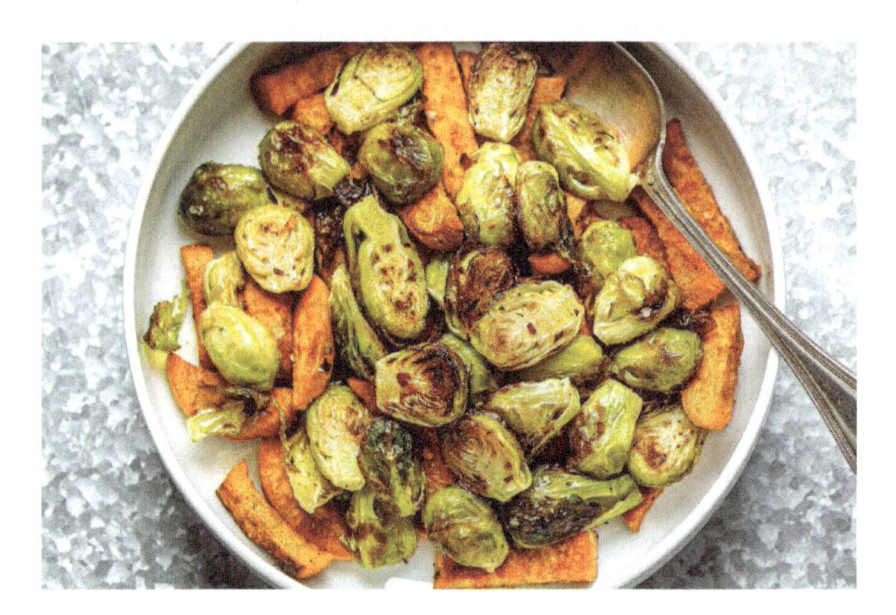

Ingredients:

- 2 medium sweet potatoes, peeled and diced
- 2 cups Brussels sprouts, halved
- 1 tablespoon olive oil
- 1/2 teaspoon garlic powder
- Salt and pepper to taste

Instructions:

Preheat the oven to 400°F.

Line a baking sheet with parchment paper.

In a large bowl, toss the sweet potatoes and Brussels sprouts with olive oil, garlic powder, salt, and pepper.

Spread the vegetables out on the prepared baking sheet.

Roast in the oven for 20-25 minutes, or until the vegetables are tender and caramelized.

Serve hot.

RECIPE 5

Chocolate Avocado Pudding

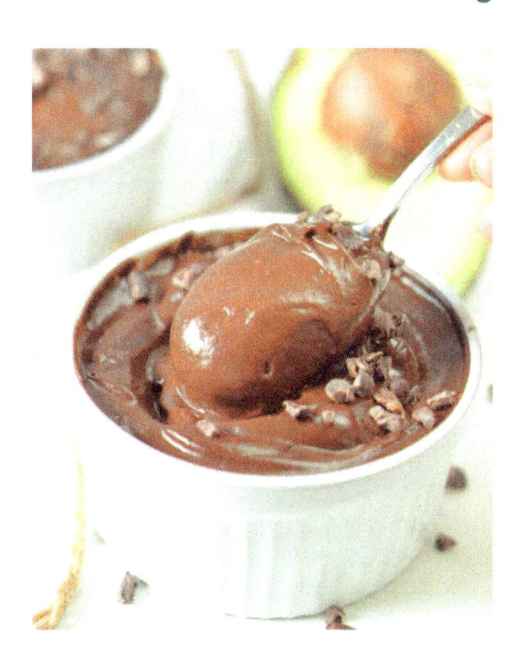

Ingredients:

- 2 ripe avocados
- 1/2 cup unsweetened cocoa powder
- 1/2 cup maple syrup
- 1/2 cup unsweetened almond milk
- 1 teaspoon vanilla extract

Instructions:

Cut the avocados in half, remove the pits, and scoop out the flesh into a blender.

Add the cocoa powder, maple syrup, almond milk, and vanilla extract.

Blend until smooth and creamy.

Pour the pudding into four individual serving dishes and chill in the refrigerator for at least 30 minutes before serving.

These hormone-balancing recipes are not only delicious but also nutrient-dense and can help support a healthy endocrine system.

EXERCISES FOR HORMONE IMBALANCES

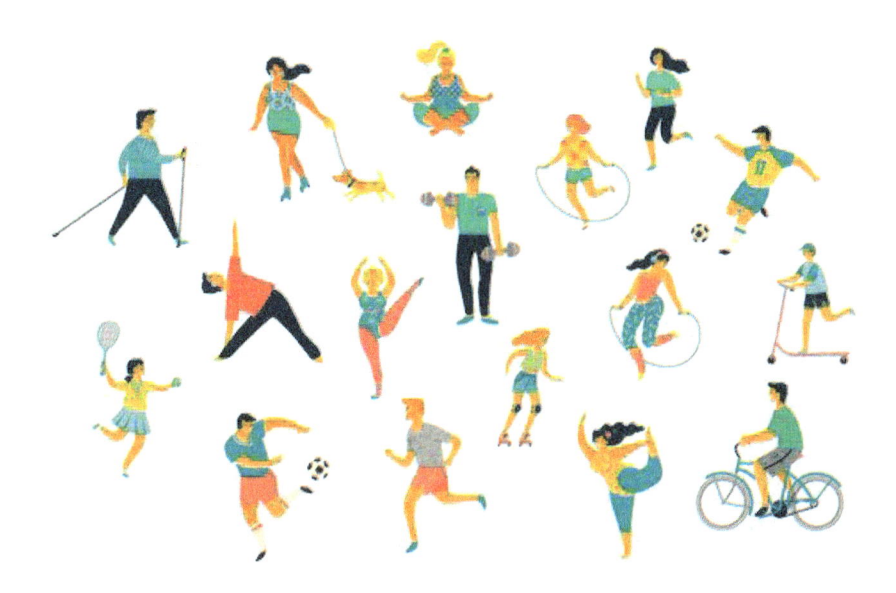

Hormone imbalances can cause various symptoms in women, such as fatigue, weight gain, mood swings, and irregular periods. Exercise is an excellent way to help manage these symptoms and support a healthy endocrine system. However, not all types of exercise are equal, and some may be more beneficial than others for women with hormone imbalances.

Walking, swimming, running, strength training, yoga, high-Intensity Interval Training, and Pilates, are all excellent forms of exercise that can improve cardiovascular health, reduce stress, and help manage symptoms of hormone imbalances in women. These exercises are low impact, making them a great option for women who may have joint pain or other limitations.

APRIL HEATH-WHITE, M.S., B.S., A.A.

Exercise Plan:

WALKING:

- Start with a 10-minute warm-up of stretching or light walking.
- Walk at a moderate pace for 30-60 minutes, depending on your fitness level.
- Cool down with 5-10 minutes of stretching or a slow walk.
- Wear comfortable shoes with good support.
- Choose a flat, even surface to walk on.
- Keep your shoulders back, relax and swing your arms naturally.
- Take deep breaths and try to maintain a steady pace.

SWIMMING:

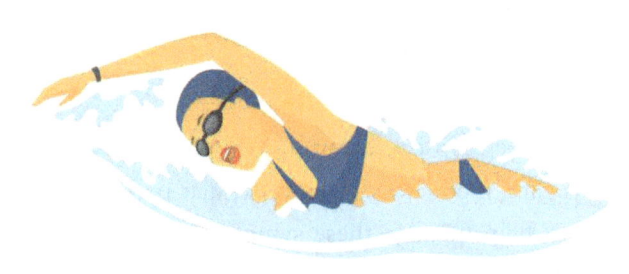

- Warm up for 5-10 minutes with some light swimming or stretching.
- Swim laps for 20-30 minutes, using a variety of strokes to work different muscle groups.
- Cool down with 5-10 minutes of slow swimming or stretching.
- Make sure you have proper swimwear and goggles.

- Start with a slow, steady pace and gradually increase your speed.
- Use a variety of strokes to work different muscle groups.
- Take breaks as needed, and drink plenty of water to stay hydrated.
- Make sure you have proper swimwear and goggles.
- Start with a slow, steady pace and gradually increase your speed.
- Use a variety of strokes to work different muscle groups.

RUNNING:

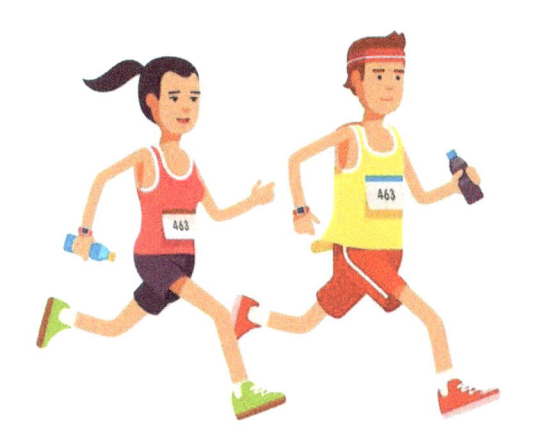

- Start with a 5–10-minute warm-up of stretching or a brisk walk.
- Run for 20-30 minutes at a moderate pace, gradually increasing your speed as your fitness level improves.
- Cool down with 5-10 minutes of walking or stretching.
- Wear comfortable, supportive running shoes.
- Choose a flat, even surface to run on.
- Start with a slow, steady pace and gradually increase your speed.

- Focus on your breathing, taking deep breaths in through your nose and out through your mouth.
- Take breaks as needed, and drink plenty of water to stay hydrated.

Note: It is important to gradually increase the intensity and duration of your workouts to avoid injury. If you are new to exercise or have any health concerns, consult with a healthcare professional before starting a new workout routine.

More Intense Exercises

Strength Training: Lifting weights or resistance bands can help build lean muscle mass and increase metabolism, improving insulin sensitivity and reducing the risk of type 2 diabetes. Strength training can also improve bone density, especially for women at risk for osteoporosis.

Yoga is a low-impact form of exercise that can reduce stress and improve mood, both of which are important for women with hormone imbalances. Certain yoga poses, such as forward folds and inversions, can stimulate the endocrine system and improve hormonal balance.

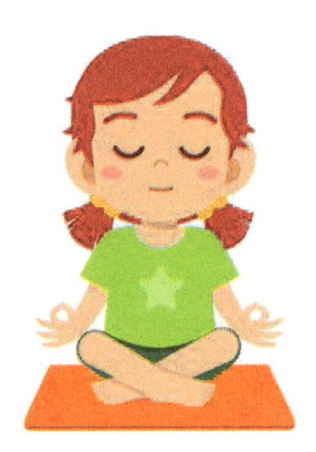

High-Intensity Interval Training (H.I.I.T.): H.I.I.T. involves short bursts of intense exercise followed by rest or low-intensity exercise periods. This type of workout can improve cardiovascular health, boost metabolism, and increase insulin sensitivity. However, women with hormone imbalances should be cautious with H.I.I.T., as excessive body stress can worsen symptoms.

Pilates: Pilates is a low-impact exercise focusing on core strength, flexibility, and balance. It can improve posture, reduce back pain, and improve overall body awareness. Pilates can also help reduce stress and improve mood, benefiting women with hormone imbalances.

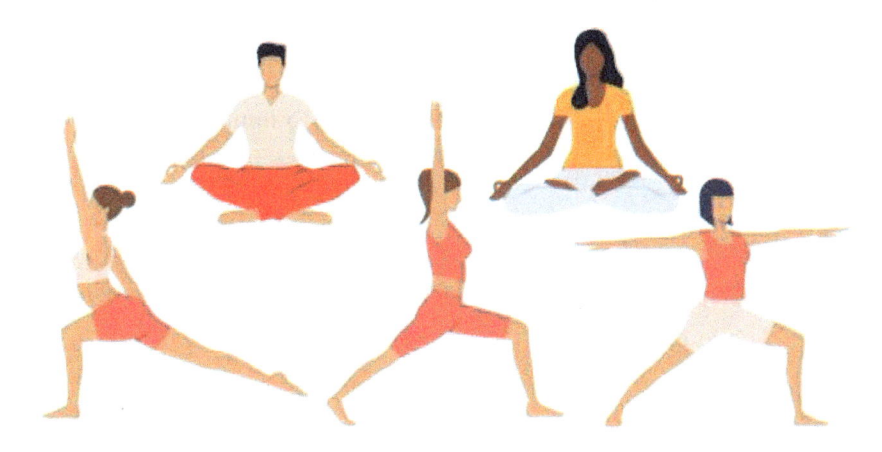

Exercise Plan:

A well-rounded exercise plan for women with hormone imbalances should include strength training, yoga, and low-impact cardio. Here is an example workout plan:

DAY 1:

- Warm-up: 5 minutes of light cardio (e.g., walking, biking, or jumping jacks)

- Strength training: 3 sets of 8-12 reps of squats, lunges, push-ups, and dumbbell rows
- Cool-down: 5 minutes of stretching

DAY 2:

- Yoga: 30-45 minutes of gentle yoga, focusing on forward folds and inversions
- Cool-down: 5 minutes of meditation or relaxation

DAY 3:

- Warm-up: 5 minutes of light cardio
- H.I.I.T.: 20 seconds of high-intensity exercise (e.g., sprinting, jumping jacks, or burpees), followed by 40 seconds of rest or low-intensity exercise. Repeat for 10-15 minutes.
- Cool-down: 5 minutes of stretching

DAY 4:

- Pilates: 30-45 minutes of Pilates, focusing on core strength and flexibility
- Cool-down: 5 minutes of stretching

Repeat this cycle for four weeks, increasing the intensity or duration of each workout as needed. Always listen to your body and modify exercises as necessary to avoid injury.

SLEEP AND HORMONE BALANCE AND HYDRATION AND HORMONE BALANCE

Getting the right amount of sleep and staying hydrated by drinking adequate water are essential to balancing hormones and maintaining overall health and well-being. Let's explore the importance of each in more detail:

Sleep and Hormone Balance:

Sleep plays a vital role in regulating hormone levels, particularly those related to stress, metabolism, appetite, and reproductive health.

Lack of sleep or poor-quality sleep can disrupt the delicate balance of hormones in the body, leading to hormone imbalances.

During sleep, the body undergoes critical therapeutic processes, including hormone synthesis, repair of tissues, and cellular rejuvenation.

Insufficient sleep can disrupt the production of hormones like cortisol, insulin, ghrelin, and leptin, which regulate energy metabolism and appetite, leading to weight gain, increased food cravings, and disrupted hunger signals.

Sleep deprivation can also impact the production of reproductive hormones, such as estrogen and progesterone, affecting menstrual regularity, fertility, and overall reproductive health.

Adequate and restful sleep helps support the optimal functioning of the endocrine system, which is responsible for hormone production and regulation.

Importance of Hydration and Hormone Balance:

Water is crucial for maintaining proper hydration, vital for overall health, and the functioning of various bodily systems, including hormone regulation.

Dehydration can disrupt hormone balance by affecting secretion, transport, and signaling.

Water transports hormones throughout the body, allowing them to reach their target organs and tissues.

Adequate hydration supports the proper functioning of the endocrine glands, which produce and release hormones into the bloodstream.

Water helps flush out toxins and waste products, promoting efficient hormone metabolism and elimination.

Proper hydration is essential for regulating body temperature, blood volume, and circulation, which can influence hormone production and distribution.

Chronic dehydration can increase stress hormone levels, electrolyte imbalances, and impaired hormone synthesis.

To balance the hormones, do these:

Aim for 7-9 hours of quality sleep each night, establishing a consistent sleep schedule and creating a conducive sleep environment.

Prioritize relaxation techniques, such as meditation, deep breathing exercises, or a calming bedtime routine, to promote better sleep quality.

Practice good sleep hygiene, including avoiding electronic devices before bed, maintaining a comfortable sleep environment, and establishing a relaxing pre-sleep routine.

Stay well-hydrated by drinking an adequate amount of water throughout the day. The general recommendation is to consume at least 8 cups (64 ounces) of water daily, but individual needs may vary based on factors such as activity level, climate, and overall health.

Back then, a beacon of hope emerged in a world where hormone imbalances wreaked havoc on women's health. It came in the form of an ancient practice known as herbal medicine. In this tale, we embark on a journey to unravel the mysteries of hormone imbalances and discover the power of herbs and natural remedies in restoring balance and vitality.

Our story's protagonist, a passionate master herbalist, who knows what it feels like to have painful periods, fibroids, and all symptoms of an imbalanced hormone, delved into the history of herbs to unlock their potential to promote hormone balance. Her quest led to uncovering the remarkable benefits of herbs like Vitex, Black cohosh, and evening primrose. Through diligent study and experimentation, she gathered evidence, case studies, and testimonials, revealing the profound impact these herbs could have on women's hormonal health.

But April did not stop there. Armed with knowledge and determination, she sought to empower women with practical tools and resources. April shared recipes, carefully crafted with ingredients and instructions, to create herbal teas, smoothies, and juices that seamlessly integrated these powerful herbs into daily routines. With each sip, women embraced the natural healing properties of these concoctions, feeling their bodies respond to the gentle touch of nature's remedies.

However, the journey to balance ended with more than herbs. April knew that exercise was vital to overall health and hormonal equilibrium. She encouraged women to embrace the joy of movement, and prescribed walks along serene paths, swims in the refreshing waters, and exhilarating runs that invigorated both body and soul.

And what about nutrition? April recognized the impact of food on hormone balance. She compiled a comprehensive list of nourishing foods, fruits, and vegetables that offered specific benefits to support hormonal health. From colorful berries bursting with antioxidants to leafy greens brimming with essential nutrients, these ingredients formed a symphony of wellness, harmonizing the intricate dance of hormones within.

April also reminded women to tread their path cautiously. She advised seeking healthcare professionals' guidance for personalized support tailored to individual needs. April urged women to stay vigilant and aware of the signs and symptoms of hormone imbalances so that early detection and intervention could pave the way to a brighter, healthier future.

As our tale draws close, the message is clear: no woman should suffer the monthly burden of hormone imbalances. With the knowledge bestowed upon her, women stood tall, embracing their power to take charge of their health. They embarked on a journey of self-care and herbal wisdom, knowing that balance and vitality awaited them on the other side.

So, to all the courageous women reading this story, remember you are capable, resilient, and have the tools to restore harmony within. Embrace the herbal way and let your hormones dance to the balanced rhythm. Your journey to wellness begins now.

THE END!

Are you a woman seeking to reclaim control over your health and well-being? Look no further; I am here to assist you on this transformative journey. As a Master Herbalist with a wealth of experience, I have dedicated myself to formulating herbal supplements and tinctures targeting hormone imbalances.

Your well-being matters to me, and I invite you to explore the wide range of services and products I offer. Whether you are interested in learning more about my expertise, purchasing herbal supplements and tinctures, or seeking guidance, I am just a click or a phone call away.

Contact me at masterherbalist@earthsgoddessholistic.com or dial 754-701-8134 to connect directly. You can also visit my website, www.earthsgoddessholistic.com, to peruse the available

herbs. Rest assured, and I am here to provide unwavering support and guidance throughout your health journey.

Every woman deserves to feel empowered, in control of her health, and harmony with her body. You will discover the tools to achieve just that through the knowledge, resources, and support offered in my book.

Thank you for joining me on this enlightening path toward wellness and balance. Your commitment to your well-being is commendable, and together, we will embark on a transformative and fulfilling adventure.

In conclusion, the art presented in this book beautifully explores the concept of balance, both in the physical and emotional realms. A harmonious equilibrium is achieved through the depiction of a balance scale and the powerful influence of herbs, specifically chaste berry, dong quai, burdock root, sea moss, dog blood, and red raspberry leaves.

The intricate artwork conveys the transformative journey of finding balance within oneself. The delicate portrayal of the balance scale symbolizes the need for equilibrium between various aspects of life, including our physical and hormonal well-being. As the pages unfold, the power of nature's remedies becomes evident, as these extraordinary herbs bring harmony to the body and mind.

Utilizing chaste berry, known for its hormone-regulating properties, alongside dong quai, burdock root, sea moss, dog blood, and red raspberry leaves, offers a holistic approach to achieving hormonal balance. The artistry captures the essence of each herb, highlighting its unique contributions to overall well-being. Through this artistic exploration, readers are invited to embrace the transformative potential of these herbs, experiencing the profound effects of hormonal balance on their lives. The art in this book serves as a visual testament to the intricate interplay between nature, human physiology, and emotional equilibrium.

Ultimately, this art collection invites us to reflect upon our journeys toward balance, encouraging us to explore the incredible healing potential of nature's gifts. May it inspire us all to cultivate harmony within ourselves and find solace in the delicate balance between body, mind, and spirit.

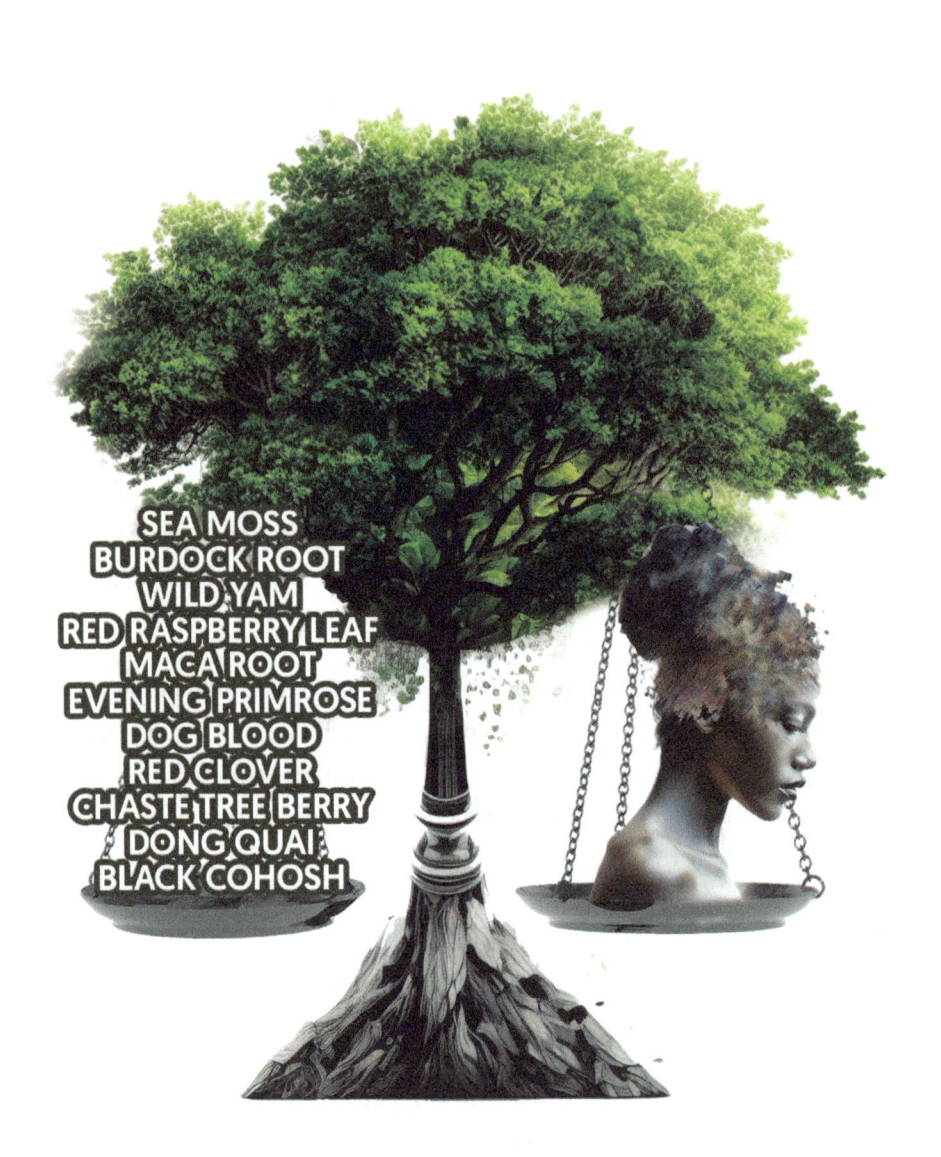

SEA MOSS
BURDOCK ROOT
WILD YAM
RED RASPBERRY LEAF
MACA ROOT
EVENING PRIMROSE
DOG BLOOD
RED CLOVER
CHASTE TREE BERRY
DONG QUAI
BLACK COHOSH